DOROTHEA OREM

Notes on Nursing Theories

SERIES EDITORS

Chris Metzger McQuiston
Doctoral Candidate, Wayne State University

Adele A. Webb
College of Nursing, University of Akron

Notes on Nursing Theories is a series of monographs designed to provide the reader with a concise description of conceptual frameworks and theories in nursing. Each monograph includes a biographical sketch of the theorist, origin of the theory, assumptions, concepts, propositions, examples for application to practice and research, a glossary of terms, and a bibliography of classic works, critiques, and research.

All monographs are available for individual purchase.

DOROTHEA OREM

Self-Care Deficit Theory

Donna L. Hartweg

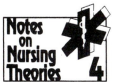

Notes
on
Nursing
Theories
4

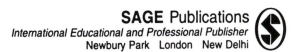

SAGE Publications
International Educational and Professional Publisher
Newbury Park   London   New Delhi

For information address:

 SAGE Publications, Inc.
2455 Teller Road
Newbury Park, California 91320
E-mail: order@sagepub.com

SAGE Publications Ltd.
6 Bonhill Street
London EC2A 4PU
United Kingdom

SAGE Publications India Pvt. Ltd.
M-32 Market
Greater Kailash I
New Delhi 110 048 India

Printed in the United States of America

Library of Congress Cataloging-in-Publication Data

Hartweg, Donna L.
    Dorothea Orem : self-care deficit theory / Donna L. Hartweg.
        p. cm. — (Notes on nursing theories ; vol. 4)
    Includes bibliographical references.
    ISBN 0-8039-4576-0 (cl) ISBN 0-8039-4299-0 (pb)
    1. Nursing — Philosophy. I Title. II. Series
    RT84.5.H37 1991
    610.73'01—dc20   91-28761
                                                                    CIP

00   01   14   13   12

Sage Production Editor: Michelle R. Starika

To Dorothea E. Orem
whose lifelong search to understand nursing has clarified
the structure of nursing knowledge and provided a foundation
for the development of a practical nursing science

Contents

Foreword

Thinking about nursing is as important as doing nursing. The conceptual structure of the discipline of nursing must be known by those nurses who practice nursing and those who teach nursing. Nurses in practice must be able to identify the phenomena that are of concern to them, and must have a framework for reflecting on their practice. The meaning given to data is a direct result of the conceptual frame the nurse brings to the practice situation. Dorothea Orem's general theory of nursing, referred to as the Self-Care Deficit Nursing Theory, provides such a framework for nurses. The elements of the theory and their elaboration in the form of propositions and descriptions provide the starting point for the development of the nurse's understanding of the conceptual framework practice.

The theory is both simple and complex. Its simplicity is found in the basic structure of the theory; its complexity in the development and implementation of those conceptual elements in practice. In order to make full use of the theory, it is necessary to comprehend the theory. This can only be done through extensive study and reflection on the original work.

This monograph complements that work, providing the reader with information about the basic structure of the theory from the viewpoint of the user. The author is well qualified to do this. She has studied the theory and has used it in teaching baccalaureate students for nearly a decade. The author draws upon this background to provide examples and interpretations, and our understanding of the theory is enhanced. As theory-based nursing becomes the norm, the expectation will be that nurses be conversant with one or more theories of nursing.

SUSAN G. TAYLOR, RN, PHD
Associate Professor,
School of Nursing,
University of Missouri-Columbia

Preface

The purpose of this volume is to present a descriptive overview of Dorothea Orem's Self-Care Deficit Theory of Nursing. It is not intended to replace the primary works of Orem, but to provide direction for their use. It is hoped that the reader will be enticed to search the writings of Orem and others for further understanding. A detailed reference list and bibliography of classic works and critiques are included to facilitate the reader's further exploration. Orem (1991), the most recent primary work at the time of this writing, is cited unless other editions or works have greater historical or substantive significance.

This book is primarily intended for use by beginning students of Orem's theory, including undergraduate students, graduate students encountering their first nursing theory course, and educators, researchers, and practitioners who are unfamiliar with Orem's work. Those familiar with the theory will find that selected chapters present a view of the Orem literature not found in other sources. For example, Chapter 1, which deals with the origins of the theory, incorporates not only the writings of Orem but also selected remarks by Orem at conferences and on videocassettes. Chapter 2 presents the assumptions, three theories, concepts, and propositions, with use of examples for clarification. Chapter 3 presents a summary of application to practice, research, and education. No attempt was made to be comprehensive, but to provide diverse examples of theory application. As this work is descriptive, no critique of Orem's work was included, although the reader should note critiques listed in the bibliography.

Teaching Orem's Self-Care Deficit Theory to undergraduate students at Illinois Wesleyan University, and subsequent doctoral study at Wayne State University, served as impetus for in-depth study of Orem's work. I am grateful to undergraduate students who challenged me to explain the theory in practical terms and to doctoral faculty who stimulated me to analyze, critique, and propose ideas and methods for theory development. My dissertation chairperson, Mary J. Denyes, served as a role model, supporting and challenging me throughout the process. The Orem Research Study group at Wayne State University provided a rich forum for further collective exploration. Self-care conferences, particularly those sponsored by the University of Missouri, have been invaluable to my own understanding and clarification. I am hopeful that this description of Orem's work will entice others to study and apply this emerging practical nursing science. I feel the product of Orem's genius is yet to be fully realized, but is indeed a means for nursing to truly make a difference in the health care of the people.

— DONNA L. HARTWEG

Acknowledgment

The author wishes to acknowledge the contribution of Susan G. Taylor, Associate Professor of Nursing, University of Missouri, Columbia, who reviewed the manuscript and made valuable suggestions for revision.

Biographical Sketch of a Nurse Theorist:
Dorothea Elizabeth Orem

Born: 1914, Baltimore, Maryland

Education: Diploma (early 1930s), Providence Hospital School of Nursing, Washington, DC; BSN Ed. (1939) and MSN Ed. (1945) from the Catholic University of America, Washington, DC.

Honorary Doctorates: Doctor of Science from Georgetown University (1976) and Incarnate Word College in San Antonio, Texas (1980); Doctor of Humane Letters from Illinois Wesleyan University, Bloomington, Illinois (1988).

Special Award: Catholic University of America Alumni Achievement Award for Nursing Theory (1980)

Current Position: Consultant in Nursing, Savannah, Georgia

1

Origin and Development

Dorothea Orem's general theory of nursing evolved over a period of four decades from individual work and through collaboration with students, practitioners, researchers, educators, administrators, and scholars. She began her work by looking for the uniqueness of nursing. How was it different from other disciplines? How was it similar? This search for distinctive nursing knowledge was directed toward answering one question, "What is the domain and what are the boundaries of nursing as a field of practice and a field of knowledge?" (Orem & Taylor, 1986, p. 39). Orem searched for the meaning of nursing, using reflection and questioning as the primary method. Today, as a consultant, Orem continues to clarify and refine her work through interaction with nurses committed to theory development. She regularly publishes new insights and gives presentations at regional, national, and international conferences.

Orem describes the model development in all primary sources. However, writings by Orem and Taylor (1986) and a video presentation, "The Nurse Theorists. Portraits of Excellence: Dorothea Orem" (Helene Fuld Health Trust, 1988), provide interesting reflections and descriptions. Eben, Gashti, Nation, Marriner-Tomey, and Nordmeyer (1989) summarize personal and professional background information based on communication and interviews with Orem.

Origins of the Model (1949-1959)

The original ideas for the model developed while Orem served as a nurse consultant with the Indiana State Board of Health between 1949 and 1957. As she traveled around the state, she became aware of the ability of nurses to do nursing, but their inability to talk about nursing. After much observation and questioning, she summarized her initial ideas about nursing in an Indiana State Board of Health report (Orem, 1956). These ideas were further developed while Orem was serving as a consultant in the Office of Education, U.S. Department of Health, Education, and Welfare. Her task was to improve the nursing component of a vocational nursing curriculum. She realized that the curriculum could not be determined until there was an understanding of the subject matter of nursing in general. Vocational nursing was a "piece of a pie" called nursing.

As a result of reflecting on her own experiences, Orem completed her search for the answer to the question, "What is nursing," through a statement about the proper object or the focus of nursing—that is, "What condition exists when judgments are made that people need nursing?" (Helene Fuld Health Trust, 1988). The answer she found was stated as follows: "The inabilities of people to care for themselves at times when they need assistance because of their state of personal health" (Orem, 1959, p. 5). This definition of nursing's focus was similar to one posed by Virginia Henderson (Henderson, 1966); however, Orem clearly stated that her own notions evolved from her unique experiences and observations, and were not derived from Henderson's work (Orem & Taylor, 1986).

Early nursing experiences that impacted Orem's ideas about nursing included practice roles of staff nurse in medical-surgical and pediatric nursing and assistant director of nursing in a general hospital. Additional positions in nursing education included those of teacher of biological sciences in a nursing program and assistant director of a school of nursing. Orem credits her ability to reflect and search for meaning in nursing both to these experiences in nursing and the study of formal logic and metaphysics, and the use of resources from many fields, including human organization and action theory. Specific literature related to action theory included the "works of Aristotle and Thomas Aquinas, as well as modern works by logicians, philosophers, psychologists, physiologists, sociologists, and industrialists" (Orem, 1987, p. 73). Important to her thinking were the works of Barnard (1962), Kotarbinski (1965), Macmurray (1957), and Parsons, Bales, and Shils (1953) (Helene Fuld Health Trust, 1988). Orem cited B. J. F. Lonergan's *Insight* (1958) as critical to her reflective thinking, and essays by Wallace (1979, 1983) as impacting more recent clarifications (Orem & Taylor, 1986). Her ideas evolved from observations in practice, with formalization coming from her extensive reading and self-reflection. Orem credits her ability to see the "whole in nursing situations" as important to her conceptualization of the theory (Helene Fuld Health Trust, 1988).

Formalization of the Model (1960-1980)

For 20 years, Orem continued to formalize her general theory of nursing with increased input from students, scholars, and colleagues. Two groups contributed significantly to the development and refinement of ideas. The Nursing Model Committee of the Nurse Faculty of The Catholic University of America, chaired by Orem, initiated its work in 1965. The impetus for the work of the committee was the inability of graduate students and faculty to identify unanswerable nursing research questions. Because the faculty identified that nursing seemed different from other disciplines, they decided to come together as a committee and develop ideas about nursing as a "mode of thought as well as a mode of doing" (Helene Fuld Health Trust, 1988).

The work of the Nursing Model Committee was continued in 1968 by the Nursing Development Conference Group (NDCG). This group was comprised of Orem and 10 other nurses with specialties in practice, education, and administration. Five of the members were from the Nursing Model Committee. The NDCG members "came together one by one because of dissatisfaction and concern due to the absence of an organizing framework for nursing knowledge and with the belief that a concept of nursing would aid in formalizing such a framework" (NDCG, 1973, p. ix). The NDCG was committed to the development of structured nursing knowledge and to nursing as a practice discipline. Group ideas refined those of Orem and formalized earlier work. This group process and the resulting product were published in two volumes, *Concept Formalization in Nursing: Process and Product*" (1973, 1979). These books, now out of print, provided rich descriptions of the work of the Nursing Development Conference Group. Other publications appeared during the decade from group members, such as Allison (1973), Backscheider (1974), and Kinlein (1977a, 1977b). Additional publications during the 1970s reflected the initial impact of Orem's work on education and practice. Piemme and Trainor (1977) described the effect of the curriculum on first-year nursing students at Georgetown University. Nowakowski (1980) described its practical application to a community-based program at Georgetown University.

Nursing: Concepts of Practice (Orem, 1971) was the original publication of the conceptual framework. A revision in 1980 presented more formalized concepts and propositions, reflecting input of the NDCG. The three theories within the general theory of nursing were an addition to the second edition. The title of the book clearly reflected Orem's practice philosophy. Concepts were developed for nursing practice to clarify the legitimate role of the nurse in practice situations. The Nursing Development Conference Group continued the emphasis on practice by using case studies to refine ideas.

Dissemination, Verification, and Current Development (1980-1991)

During the 1980s, Orem revised *Nursing: Concepts of Practice* (1985b). Changes were limited to the addition of assumptions and definitions of selected concepts, such as health. The fourth edition, published in 1991, included several substantive changes, such as new propositions in the Theory of Self-Care. Additionally, selected components of *Concept Formalization in Nursing: Process and Product* (1979) not previously included in *Nursing: Concepts of Practice* (1971, 1980, 1985b), were integrated throughout the book.

Clarification of components in the model continued throughout the decade, partially in response to analysis and critiques of the theory. For example, Meleis (1985) questioned the model's utility in promoting health and well-being. Hartweg (1990) subsequently described a conceptualization of health promotion self-care within the model. Health promotion self-care was defined as self-care to promote well-being rather than health as a physical and functional state. Orem (1985b) defined health as the integrity of human structure and functioning. In contrast, well-being was described as happiness, contentment, and fulfillment of one's self-ideal. Hartweg viewed this clarification of health promotion self-care as a necessary step for specific health promotion self-care practice and research.

The decade was also one of increased application, testing, and refinement through nursing practice and research (see Chapter 3). As numerous scholars, educators, researchers, practitioners, and administrators encountered the model, communication became essential. Dr. Susan Taylor, University of Missouri, Columbia, facilitated dissemination through initiation of a *Self-Care Deficit Theory Curriculum Network Directory* (1980) and later as newsletter coordinator of the *Self-Care Deficit Nursing Theory Newsletter* (available through the School of Nursing, University of Missouri, Columbia). With Taylor's leadership, the University of Missouri, Columbia, began sponsoring biannual conferences in 1982 that facilitated communication and promoted development of selected concepts. For example, the Sixth Annual Self-Care Deficit Theory Conference, held in 1987, examined two concepts within the model, nursing agency and nursing systems. Work sessions were held with scholars, practitioners, and researchers who shared ideas regarding concept development. Proceedings of the conferences were published. Other conferences were held regularly in Toronto, Ontario, and Vancouver, British Columbia. The First International Self-Care Deficit Nursing Theory (S-CDNT) Conference was held in Kansas City in 1989, with participants from Sweden, Netherlands, Canada, Thailand, Australia, Japan, and the United States. This participation reflected the global impact of the theory. Examples of the international application and development of the model are included throughout Chapter 3.

In addition to conferences, scholarly groups developed in institutions. An Orem Research Study Group was organized in 1984 at Wayne State University, Detroit, MI. Doctoral students and faculty regularly meet to facilitate model development and testing. Publications have resulted from the group's work (Denyes, O'Connor, Oakley, & Ferguson, 1989; Gast et al. 1989).

During this period, journals increasingly focused on articles about the theory. Fawcett (1989) provided a detailed summary of articles and personal communications on its application and utilization in practice, education, research, and administration. Examples of application included all clinical areas and nursing settings. Numerous articles appeared in international journals (e.g., Rosenbaum, 1989). Orem was named to an advisory panel for *Nursing Science Quarterly: Theory, Research, and Practice*. Theory-based computer software for bedside care was developed within Orem's general theory of nursing by Nursing Systems International. The Self-Care model linked the patient assessments with nursing diagnosis, expected patient outcomes, discharge planning, quality assurance variables, clinical research, and external agency reports.

Future Directions for Theory Development

Continued development will distinguish among variations in the concepts, develop rules for nursing practice, and finally establish rules for nursing specific populations. Orem dreams of a time when a general theory of nursing is no longer needed, but replaced by practice models and rules specific to populations and subgroups in need of nursing (Orem, 1988, November). Orem (1987, 1988) proposed future directions by identifying five stages for model development. Stage one includes the development of the theory, with identification of the concepts and their relationships. This stage has been completed. Stage two is an investigation of variations in nursing situations. The development and testing of the concept of self-care agency in various populations and settings is an example of this stage, which is in progress. Stage three is the development of models and rules for nursing practice. Examples of such models include those by Horn and Swain (1977), who created standards for determining nursing's effectiveness, and the preliminary work by Orem (1984, 1985b) on application to families and communities. Stage four includes the development of nursing cases by practitioners within the nursing model. Some case studies are now recorded (Orem & Taylor, 1986), but many others need to be observed and recorded. Stage five is the development of models and rules for providing nursing to populations. Orem suggests this includes nursing provided to entire populations, such as those in a hospital. She views this as important to nursing administration and nursing economics. Stages three, four, and five need much development.

The stages suggested by Orem for model development clearly reflect her beliefs about the importance of nursing practice. She believes that this development will facilitate the understanding of nursing as a "practical science" (Orem, 1988).

2

Assumptions, Theories, Concepts, and Propositions

Orem's theory has been called a general theory of nursing, Self-Care Deficit Theory of Nursing, Self-Care Deficit Nursing Theory, and Self-Care Theory of Nursing. Orem (1980) described her work as a general theory of nursing comprising three "articulating" or interrelated theories: theory of self-care, theory of self-care deficit, and theory of nursing systems. The specific name for Orem's general theory of nursing however, is Self-Care Deficit Theory of Nursing, or S-CDTN (Orem, 1991). She chose the name "deficit" as it describes and explains a relationship between abilities of individuals to care for themselves and the self-care needs or demands of the individual, their children, or the adults for whom they care. The notion of "deficit" does not refer to a specific type of limitation, but to the relationship between the capabilities of the individual and the needs for action. Although Orem focuses on the individual throughout the major works, the model can be used with families (Orem, 1983b, 1983c; Tadych, 1985; Taylor, 1989), and communities (Orem, 1984; Hanchett, 1988, 1990).

Assumptions in Self-Care Deficit Theory of Nursing

Orem (1991) described several sets of assumptions. The first and most basic are general assumptions that relate to the entire general theory of nursing. There are also assumptions that Orem called presuppositions, which relate to each of the three interrelated theories. Assumptions are also identified that relate to specific concepts, such as the concept of self-care requisites. These assumptions throughout S-CDTN serve to guide thinking about the many component parts of the theory.

Five general assumptions or generalizations about human beings relate to all three theories and have been implicit in Orem's thinking from the beginning. These "principles of nursing," as she called them in the early years, were initially presented in 1973 in a paper given by Orem at the Fifth Annual Post-Masters Conference of Marquette University's School of Nursing (Orem, 1987). They were not published until 1985 in *Nursing: Concepts of Practice*. More recently, she referred to the five assumptions as the underlying premises of the general theory (Orem, 1991, pp. 66-67).

These premises or general assumptions about individual human beings, their capabilities and their relationships, provided an important foundation for the future development of specific concepts of the general theory. For example, two assumptions that describe human agency were important to the later development of the concepts of self-care agency and nursing agency. These assumptions describe the relationship of requirements for human action (demand) and human agency, as well as the sociocultural basis for nursing.

Three Interrelated Theories

Each of the interrelated theories of self-care, self-care deficit, and nursing systems has a central idea, a set of propositions and presuppositions (Orem, 1991, pp. 67-73). The central idea describes the focus of the theory. The set of propositions are statements that describe concepts or relationships among concepts in the theory; refer to Table 2.2 for a list of propositions. Presuppositions are assumptions, or "givens," that are more specific to each of the three theories than the general assumptions. Orem explained that these sets of presuppositions help link the three theories to one another. For example, Set One of the presuppositions under the theory of self-care deficit (or dependent-care deficit) provides the link to the theory of self-care. Set Two links the theory of self-care deficit to the theory of nursing system. Orem (1987) also identified specific questions to be addressed by each theory.

Theory of Self-Care Deficit (or Dependent-Care Deficit)

The central idea, six propositions, and two sets of presuppositions in the theory of self-care deficit (Orem, 1991, pp. 70-71) propose an answer to the question, "When and why do people require the health service nursing?" (Orem, 1987, p. 72). The central idea is that individuals are affected from time to time by limitations that do not allow them to meet their self-care needs. These limitations may occur because of a health condition, such as an accident or diabetes, or because of factors that are internal or external to the individual. For example, an internal factor is age. Certain self-care limitations may occur with age, such as those of a geriatric client, that place the person in need of nursing. An example of an external factor is a specific life experience, such as an unexpected death in the family. This event may incapacitate a person and limit the ability to meet general or specific human needs. Orem is clear that nursing must be "legitimate"—that is, the relationship between the person-nurse and the person-patient is based on the condition that establishes a need for nursing and not some other condition such as a medical condition.

Theory of Self-Care (Dependent-Care)

The central idea, six propositions, and four presuppositions in the theory of self-care (Orem, 1991, pp. 69-70) propose to answer the question, "What is self-care and what is dependent care?" (Orem, 1987, p. 72). Orem (1991) made substantive changes in the propositions of this theory, replacing 10 principles with 6 new propositions.

Two ideas about self-care are emphasized in the theory: self-care as learned behavior and self-care as deliberate action. Self-care is described as behavior that is learned from interaction and communication in larger social groups. A presupposition is that self-care actions vary by the cultural and social experiences of the individual. In other words, the self-care actions performed in response to needs created by respiratory illness will vary among individuals who have been raised in different social or cultural environments. Cao gio, or coin rubbing, is a self-care action learning within the Vietnamese culture and initiated in response to respiratory illness (Hautman, 1987). Self-care and dependent care are performed "purposively," or with purpose. A related phrase throughout the theory is "deliberate action." Self-care is not instinctive or reflexive, but performed rationally in response to a known need. One such need for women that is known through our knowledge of medical science is to perform breast self-examination. Some women will take deliberate action to gain the knowledge and subsequently perform the action every month. Other women will not seek the knowledge or take action. Orem explains this through two presuppositions. All individuals have the potential ability and motivation necessary to provide care for themselves and dependents. However, having the ability or potential does not mean that all will seek knowledge or take action.

Dependent care is explained indirectly though the theory of self-care. Orem (1991) states that self-care is performed by mature and maturing individuals. If self-care is learned and performed deliberately in response to a need, it assumes that the individual has had time for interaction and communication to learn about the necessary action. It also assumes that the physical and intellectual development are present to perform the action. But self-care cannot be performed if the abilities have not had time to develop and mature, or if developed abilities have become inoperable. Infants and children cannot meet the requirements necessary for life, health, and well-being because they are not developed. Adults who have matured and developed are at times unable to met their needs. The abilities of a 20-year-old comatose, motorcycle accident victim have developed over time. But because of a comatose state, the abilities are not "operable"—that is, the patient cannot use that which has been learned. In these situations where all or some abilities are underdeveloped and inoperable, someone must perform the self-care. When a family member or responsible adult performs such care, it is termed "dependent care."

Theory of Nursing System

Understanding Orem's theory of nursing system is the key to understanding her general theory of nursing. The major components of the theory of self-care and the theory of self-care deficit are incorporated within the theory of nursing system (Orem & Taylor, 1986). Orem (1987) therefore called this the "unifying theory." The "theory of nursing system subsumes the theory of self-care deficit, which subsumes the theory of self-care" (Orem, 1991, p. 66). It is through this theory that the relationship between nursing actions and role and patient actions and role are explained. The central idea, eight propositions, and two presuppositions propose an answer to three questions: "What do nurses do when they nurse?" "What is the product made by nurses?" and "What results are sought by nurses?" (Orem, 1987, p. 72). These questions are similar to the questions that guided Orem's initial development of the general theory and provide understanding of why she views it as the unifying theory.

The central idea is that nurses have abilities that they use to determine if nursing help is necessary or "legitimate." The process involves the nurse determining an existing or potential deficit relationship between the abilities and demands for action in situations involving the health of an individual. If the deficit relationship exists, then the nurse should design a plan of care that clearly identifies what is to be done and by whom: the nurse, the patient, or the family member. These actions of the nurse and of the patient and/or dependent-care giver are collectively called the nursing system. The goal of the nursing system is to increase the patient's capabilities to meet a need, or requisite, or to decrease the demand. The two presuppositions assume that nursing is a practical service that has its own domain and boundaries. It is composed of deliberate actions over a period of time. If a nurse is performing an injection in a doctor's office as a one-time function, a nursing system for that patient may not be developed unless the nurse and patient together determine that follow-up on the injection or further nursing intervention is necessary.

Summary

The three theories of self-care, self-care deficit, and nursing system are interrelated through the presuppositions. Researchers and practitioners select one or all of the theories to guide their work. However, sometimes nurses focus their care primarily within one theory. For example, a nurse in an acute care setting may use the theory of self-care deficit, while the nurse in an ambulatory care setting may function primarily within the theory of self-care (Taylor, 1990). However, the key to understanding is through the theory of nursing systems, which describes and explains the nursing role.

Concepts

S-CDTN is composed of six basic concepts and one related, or peripheral, concept. The basic, or core, concepts are self-care, self-care agency, therapeutic self-care demand, self-care deficit, nursing agency, and nursing system. The concepts of self-care, self-care agency, therapeutic self-care demand, and self-care deficit are related to the patient, or the person in need of nursing, while the concepts of nursing agency and nursing system are related to the nurses and their actions. The concept of basic conditioning factors is related to selected patient and nurse concepts. Within the set of patient concepts, basic conditioning factors relate to self-care agency and to therapeutic self-care demand. Within the set of nurse concepts, they relate to nursing agency. Basic conditioning factors influence selected concepts. These include "age, gender, developmental state, health state, sociocultural orientation, health care system factors . . . family system factors, pattern of living, . . . environmental factors, resource availability and adequacy" (Orem, 1991, p. 136). Additional conditioning factors, such as nursing educational preparation and nursing experience, influence nursing agency. (See Figure 2.1.)

The assumptions, definitions, and relationships of each of the concepts are presented below. Historical context is presented where relevant.

Self-Care (Dependent Care)

Orem defines self-care as "the practice of activities that individuals initiate and perform on their own behalf in maintaining life, health, and well-being" (Orem, 1991, p. 117). This definition has been used consistently since the earliest descriptions of self-care by Orem (1956; 1959).

The general assumptions about self-care evolved from Orem's original papers and through the work of the Nursing Model Committee and the Nursing Development Conference Group (NDCG). Members of the groups spent 2 years clarifying the concept through analysis of specific practice situations and through subsequent validation of self-care conduct through group analysis of case study films (NDCG, 1973).

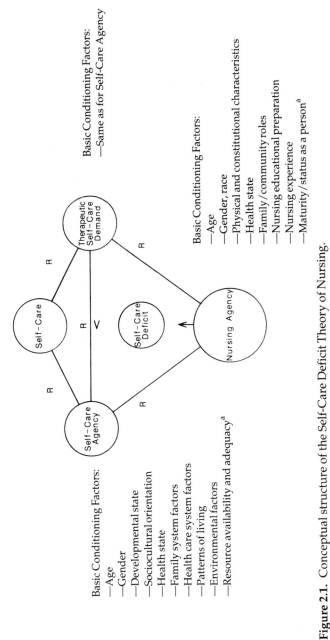

Figure 2.1. Conceptual structure of the Self-Care Deficit Theory of Nursing.

SOURCE: Adapted from Orem, 1987, p. 70, by permission of W. B. Saunders

a. Orem, 1991

NOTES: R = relationship; < means that a self-care deficit exists when self-care agency is less than the therapeutic self-care demand

Basic assumptions of the concept that have been consistent throughout development of the model include the following: (a) self-care is ego-processed activity, which is learned through the individual's interpersonal relations and communications; (b) each adult person has both the right and responsibility to care for self; this may include responsibilities for others, such as infants, children, the aged, or an adolescent; and (c) an adult may need assistance from time to time to accomplish self-care (NDCG, 1973, p. 99). Self-care is not assumed to contribute to the positive nature of the health state. However, it is assumed that at the time when the individual first selected and performed the self-care action, it was done with the understanding that it was related in some way to health or well-being (NDCG, 1973).

Orem refers to self-care as "deliberate action." As learned behavior, it is goal directed with a purpose in mind. A person consumes water, knowing that life and health cannot continue without it. A person with hypertension takes prescribed medication, knowing its importance in maintaining blood pressure within a healthy range. A 50-year-old woman increases the intake of calcium in her diet, knowing its importance in the prevention of osteoporosis in later life. Each of these instances is an example of a learned, goal-directed self-care action in which the prerequisite of "knowing" and "deciding" is presented. This emphasizes that self-care has phases. To perform a self-care action for a specific purpose one must first have knowledge of the action and how it relates to continued life, health, or well-being. The woman must seek and find information about the special calcium needs of middle-aged women and then reflect on the information. She then must make a decision either to change her food habits to obtain additional calcium or not to change food habits to meet the increased calcium needs for middle-aged women. These phases of seeking knowledge and decision making must precede the obvious self-care action of consuming or not consuming selected foods with increased calcium. Therefore one self-care action is composed of a series of operations, or phases. The early development of two series was developed by Backscheider (1974) and Pridham (1971). The phases of self-care are described by Orem (1991) as estimative, transitional, and productive operations. The phases of deliberate action are detailed by Orem (p. 85), with subsequent elaboration of phases of the three types of operations (pp. 85, 163-167).

The related concept of dependent care is within definitions of self-care. Dependent care is "actions performed by responsible adults to meet the components of their dependents' therapeutic self-care demands" (Orem & Taylor, 1986, p. 49). Orem is clear that the focus in dependent care given by families, friends, or other adults to other persons is related to the dependent's inability to provide the care needed because of a health state and not because of needs related to age or development (Orem, 1985b). That is to say, the term dependent care is not used for the normal care provided by a mother to her infant. But when the needs of the child change due to health state, such as an episode of pneumonia, then dependent care becomes relevant.

Self-Care Agency (Dependent-Care Agency)

Orem describes self-care agency as the power of individuals to engage in self-care and capability for self-care (NDCG, 1979, p. 181). The person who uses this power or self-care ability is the self-care agent. Assumptions about self-care agency (p. 183) are inherent in these definitions. Self-care agency is an acquired ability that is affected by conditions and factors in the environment. For example, an individual who is educationally deprived may have less ability to seek information about health care than one who has had many educational opportunities. Self-care agency is an ability to engage in self-care that develops from childhood, reaches maturity in adulthood, and declines with old age. Dependent-care agency is the ability of responsible adults to meet the continuing demands for self-care of their dependents.

Self-care agency, as a theoretical concept, has evolved from the early work of the NDCG as power and ability. It is described as a complex, hierarchical three-part structure (Orem & Taylor, 1986); see Figure 2.2. As one progresses from the base upward, the components relate more specifically to abilities needed for specific self-care action.

Part 1: Foundational Capabilities and Dispositions. The base of the structure includes the foundational capabilities and dispositions necessary for persons to engage in all types of deliberate action, not only self-care. For example, an individual may "deliberately act" to fix the car. Foundational capabilities are necessary, such as ability to work, to regulate position and movement of the body, and to remember directions for the repair. Dispositions affecting the goal of the action are also required, such as awareness of one's ability to make the repairs. Other capabilities and dispositions are components of this foundation, such as interests and values of the individual (NDCG, 1979, p. 212).

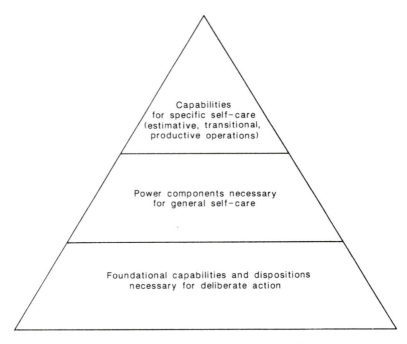

Figure 2.2. The three-part hierarchical structure of self-care agency.
SOURCE: Adapted from Gast et al., 1989, p. 27, by permission of Aspen Publishers, Inc., © 1989

Part 2: Power Components. Ten power components comprise the middle portion of the hierarchy and relate specifically to self-care (see Table 2.1). Capabilities, such as motivation to engage in self-care, are clearly necessary for the individual to take action. To perform self-care, these "empowering capabilities" for self-care must be developed and operating. If a patient is comatose, the ability to maintain attention is not present. The ability may have been developed over time, but is clearly not operating at the present. In the absence of the operability of self-care agency, nursing or dependent-care agents will need to provide compensatory care. Orem states that the 10 power components can be summarized as knowledge, attitudes, and skills that enable the individual to engage in self-care (Orem, 1990).

Part 3: Capabilities for Estimative, Transitional, and Productive Operations. The level in the hierarchy closest to the concrete self-care action is

TABLE 2.1 Power Components of Self-Care Agency

1. Ability to maintain attention and exercise requisite vigilance with respect to (a) self as self-care agent and (b) internal and external conditions and factors significant to self-care

2. Controlled use of available physical energy that is sufficient for the initiation and continuation of self-care operations

3. Ability to control the position of the body and its part in the execution of the movements required for the initiation and completion of self-care operations

4. Ability to reason within a self-care frame of reference

5. Motivation (i.e., goal orientations for self-care that are in accord with its characteristics and its meaning for life, health, and well-being)

6. Ability to make decisions about care of self and to operationalize these decisions

7. Ability to acquire technical knowledge about self-care from authoritative sources, to retain it, and operationalize it

8. A repertoire of cognitive, perceptual, manipulative, communication, and interpersonal skills adapted to the performance of self-care operations

9. Ability to order discrete self-care actions or action systems into relationships with prior and subsequent actions toward the final achievement of regulatory goals of self-care

10. Ability to consistently perform self-care operations, integrating them with relevant aspects of personal, family, and community living

SOURCE: Reprinted from Nursing Development Conference Group, *Concept Formalization: Process and Product*, 1979, pp. 195-196, by permission of Little, Brown, and Company.

composed of three specific types of power and abilities: the ability to determine what needs to be done to regulate one's health and well-being; ability to judge and decide what to do from the information that has been obtained; and the ability to actually perform the self-care actions once the knowledge is obtained and the decision to act has been made. These three capabilities are related to three types of action necessary to meet specific self-care demands: estimative, transitional, and productive operations or actions, respectively (NDCG, 1979; Orem, 1991). Estimative actions are those the individual performs when determining what self-care is to be performed; that is, the 50-year-old woman reads books and asks her nurse practitioner or physician about the special calcium needs of middle-aged women. Transitional operations or actions include reflecting on the course of action to be taken and then making a decision. The middle-aged woman must reflect on a variety of options related to the need for calcium. Should she change her daily food habits to obtain additional calcium or maintain the same food habits and consume calcium tablets daily? Productive operations relate to preparing the self to add this new self-care action to the daily routine, monitoring the effects of the new self-care action, and deciding the effectiveness of the action. If the middle-aged woman decides to take calcium tablets, productive operations would include purchasing the tablets, integrating the action into the daily routine, and determining their effect on her health and well-being. Specific abilities are necessary for each of these three types of actions.

Although the complexity of the concept was apparent in the early work, efforts to develop instruments to measure self-care agency have revealed its many dimensions or elements (Gast et al. 1989). Orem (1987) refers to self-care agency as the "summation of all the human capabilities needed for performing self-care" (p. 76) in actual situations. It combines those necessary for deliberate action, those required for general self-care, and those relevant to specific self-care.

Therapeutic Self-Care Demand

Therapeutic self-care demand (TSCD) is a concept that developed from the work of the NDCG over a 3-year period. It can be thought of as a collection of actions to be performed, or a "program of action" (NDCG, 1979, p. 184). It addresses this question: What are *all* the self-care actions that *should be performed* by the individual over time to maintain life, health, and well-being? Orem (1991) more recently described these as the "summation of measures of self-care required at moments in time and for some duration" (p. 65). This summation or totality of care actions is performed to meet what Orem calls self-care requisites, or generalized purposes for which the individual performs self-care. The self-care requisite is the general purpose. For example, a person deliberately drinks a quantity of water each day to maintain a sufficient intake of water, a basic self-care requisite. When a person deliberately selects and eats food, the self-care action is meeting the requisite for "maintenance of sufficient intake of food."

Each individual has only one therapeutic self-care demand that must be calculated from extensive knowledge and skill to meet the many known requirements or requisites that promote life, health, and well-being. Through experience, the individual learns about the specific requirements that must be met. As new events occur, such as illness or pregnancy, health care workers inform the individual of new requirements for action. Therefore there is an interlinking of scientific knowledge and knowledge inherent within the person and the environment (NDCG, 1979).

Orem identified three types of self-care requisites, or requirements, for action: universal, developmental, and health deviation. Universal self-care requisites are those of all human beings throughout all stages of the life cycle, and can be adjusted for age, environment, and other factors. There are eight universal self-care requisites:

1. The maintenance of sufficient intake of air.
2. The maintenance of a sufficient intake of water.
3. The maintenance of a sufficient intake of food.
4. The provision of care associated with elimination processes and excrements.
5. The maintenance of a balance between activity and rest.
6. The maintenance of a balance between solitude and social interaction.
7. The prevention of hazards to human life, human functioning, and human well-being.
8. The promotion of human functioning and development within social groups in accord with human potential, known human limitations, and the human desire to be normal. *Normalcy* is used in the sense of that which is essentially human and that which is in accord with the genetic and constitutional characteristics and the talents of individuals.[1]

Normalcy relates to the development of a realistic self-concept. Developmental self-care requisites are of two types, the first being maturational and related to the universals, but adjusted for age or developmental stage. For example, needs for food and interaction in adulthood are different from needs for food and interaction as a neonate. The second type of developmental requisite is situational and related to self-care that prevents or overcomes effects of life events or experiences that can impact human development. Examples include the tragedy of death, a change of residence, or those experiences related to social conditions, such as educational deprivation or oppressive living conditions. Each of these creates new requirements that must be met by the individual for life, health, and well-being.

Six health deviation self-care requisites exist for individuals who are "ill, are injured, have specific forms of pathology including defects and disabilities, and who are under medical diagnosis and treatment" (Orem, 1991, p. 132). Both genetic and acquired defects from health and well-being bring about needs for actions to prevent further problems or to control and overcome the effects of the existing deviations from normal. Because knowledge of these conditions emanates from medical science and technology, many of these needs are not known by individuals and must be learned through interaction with health care professionals. For example, the first health deviation self-care requisite cited by Orem suggests a need for women at risk for breast cancer, an example of "evidence of genetic conditions known to produce pathology" (p. 134), to seek assistance to learn self-breast examination and to seek resources and monitoring through mammography. The frequency of such self-care actions may be different from those who are not at risk.

Ideal sets of actions to be taken by patients with specific health conditions are being identified and are forming the basis for assessment in health care institutions where Orem's model is being used as the framework for practice. For example, ideal sets of actions have been identified for patients with laryngectomies and angina (Harry S. Truman Veteran's Administration, 1986, p. 131).

The ability to "calculate" all the self-care actions to be performed to meet all the universal, developmental, and health deviation self-care requisites requires much knowledge about health, illness, and human development. In addition, it requires much information about individuals and groups, including specific cultures. Orem is clear that the therapeutic self-care demand or component of self-care demand must be known before the individual can engage in self-care. Once the requirements are known, then the adequacy of self-care agency can be assessed in relationship to the known self-care demand. It is, therefore, the TSCD that is much like a standard and "sets the specifications for self-care agency as well as for self-care" (NDCG, 1979, p. 181).

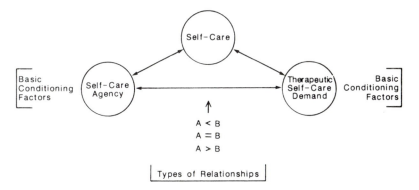

Figure 2.3. The three types of relationships between self-care agency
and therapeutic self-care demand.
SOURCE: Adapted from Orem, 1991, p. 146, by permission of Mosby-Year Book, Inc.

Self-Care Deficit (Dependent-Care Deficit)

Self-care deficit is a patient-focused concept that expresses a qualitative and quantitative relationship between two concepts, self-care
agency and therapeutic self-care demand. There are three possible
relationships: greater than, equal to, or less than/not adequate (see
Figure 2.3).

A self-care deficit is the "relationship between self-care agency and
therapeutic self-care demands of individuals in which capabilities for
self-care, because of existent limitations, are not equal to meeting some
or all of the components of their therapeutic self-care demands"
(Orem, 1991, p. 173). A dependent care deficit is an unequal relationship between capabilities (agency) of responsible adults and the dependent person's required therapeutic self-care demand. A self-care
deficit or dependent-care deficit may exist with a current inadequacy
or may be predicted for the future as changes in either self-care agency
(dependent-care agency) or therapeutic self-care demand are antici-
pated (Orem, 1987). Orem is clear that the deficit itself is not a disorder
or problem, but an expression of this relationship between the two
concepts. This self-care deficit, or potential for a self-care deficit, must
exist for nursing to be legitimate. If the nurse and the patient determine
that no current or potential self-care deficit exists, then there is no role
for the nurse in this situation.

Self-care deficit is a conceptual element and is described as complete or partial—that is, after determining the sum of all self-care actions necessary to meet the requisites (the therapeutic self-care demand), and an assessment of the adequacy of self-care agency in relationship to the therapeutic self-care demand, the nurse can determine whether a self-care deficit exists and whether it is partial or complete. A complete self-care deficit means "no capability to meet a therapeutic self-care demand" (Orem, 1991, p. 173). A partial deficit exists when the individual has some capabilities to meet part of the therapeutic self-care demand, but not all. A mother with an infant has the capability to carry out most of the self-care actions to meet universal self-care requisites, but may need assistance with new developmental demands, such as care of breasts if she is breastfeeding.

Nursing Agency

Nursing agency, or collective nursing capabilities, is defined as the "complex property or attribute of persons educated and trained as nurses that is enabling when exercised for knowing and helping others know their therapeutic self-care demands, for helping others meet or in meeting their therapeutic self-care demands, and in helping others regulate the exercise or development of their self-care agency or their dependent-care agency" (Orem, 1991, p. 64). This theoretical concept has a three-part structure similar to self-care agency (refer to Figure 2.2). There are also necessary foundational capabilities and dispositions, such as positive attitudes and willingness to act. The power components of nursing agency are similar to self-care agency, but are specific to providing nursing, such as motivation to provide nursing care and the ability to control body parts as developed nursing skills. The third and most specific capabilities include those necessary for steps of the nursing process, such as diagnosis, prescription, and regulation or development of the person's self-care agency, or meeting of the therapeutic self-care demand (Orem & Taylor, 1986). Within these specialized abilities, Orem (1991) identified three types of desired nursing characteristics: social, interpersonal, and technological (pp. 261-263). These characteristics suggest the need for knowledge and skill that includes not only specific nursing knowledge, but also a strong foundation in the humanities, sciences, and arts.

Like self-care agency, nursing agency is a complex, acquired ability of adults to engage in deliberate action; that is, it is learned and performed

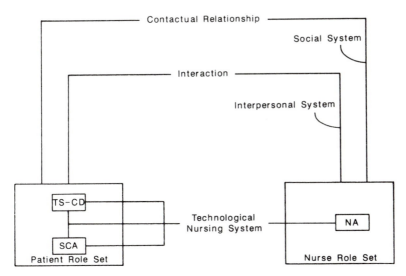

Figure 2.4. A hierarchy of interlocking systems.
SOURCE: Reprinted from Nursing Development Conference Group, 1979, p. 112, by permission of Little, Brown and Company, © 1979
NOTE: TS-CD=therapeutic self-care demand; SCA= self-care agency; NA= nursing agency

with a goal in mind. It is specialized ability that varies in nurses through their educational experiences, their practice situations, their mastery of skills, and their ability to work with and care for others (Orem, 1985b). Capabilities of a new graduate nurse will differ from those of an experienced clinician. Orem (1991) elaborated on other factors important to the ultimate delivery of nursing care. Factors such as age, gender, race, culture, status, and maturity as a person may affect the relations with patients. The focus of nursing agency differs from self-care agency as follows: Nursing agency is "developed and exercised for the benefit and well-being of others and self-care agency is developed and exercised for the benefit and well-being of oneself" (Orem, 1991, p. 255).

Orem (1985b) described nursing agency as "activated or un-activated." Activated agency produces diagnosis, prescription, and regulation of self-care for persons with self-care deficits associated with their health state. When nursing agency is activated as such, a nursing system is produced.

Nursing System

Orem (1985b) defined nursing system generally as "all the actions and interactions of nurses and patients in nursing practice situations" (p. 148). This concept emerged from the early work of the Nursing Model Committee of Catholic University in 1970 as the "creative end product of nursing" (NDCG, 1973, p. 69). More recently, Orem (1991) described the concept as "something constructed through actions of nurses and nurses' patients . . . a product that should be beneficial to persons with patient status in nursing practice situations when the time frame for production fits the time of occurrence of requirements for nursing" (p. 63).

Nursing system is viewed as tridimensional, including a hierarchy of interlocking systems: social, interpersonal, and technological (see Figure 2.4). The social and interpersonal dimensions are common to all helping services. The technological dimension is specific to nursing and gives direction to the form and substance of nursing. It is within this component that the elements of therapeutic self-care demand, self-care agency, and nursing agency are interrelated. The efforts of the nurse are directed toward the "ability of others to engage in self-care effectively and continuously and . . . the continuous and effective meeting of the existing self-care requisites of others in the event of health-derived or health-related self-care deficits" (Orem, 1985b, pp. 147-148). However, Figure 2.4 clarifies assumptions of Orem and the NDCG that social and interpersonal aspects of nursing are also essential to the nursing system.

The social system is considered enabling of the interpersonal and technological systems (NDCG, 1973). The social system must exist or there is no basis for establishing the interpersonal relationship. The social system clarifies the role of the person as patient and the role of the nurse as the provider of care. If a self-care deficit exists, the person may become a patient of the nurse. If a person has nursing agency and the willingness to provide helping methods, a person may become the nurse of the patient. However, a critical element is also necessary: the establishment of a contractual relationship within the social system. This includes a contract or a formal agreement that clarifies the boundaries of the nursing care, the length of time for the care, and remuneration for the care. In such institutions as hospitals, this agreement may be implied when the patient signs an admission contract for care by nurses who are employed by the institution. Orem (1985b) emphasized the importance of the contractual nature of nurse-patient relationships in the following statement: "If nurses would accept the purpose of nursing and the contractual nature of nursing relationships, the deleterious practices of viewing patients as objects to be acted on and of processing patients through a system of routinized measures regardless of their conditions and needs might be eliminated" (p. 226).

Two factors produce the necessary interaction that occurs between the nurse and the patient in the interpersonal system: contact and association. The notion of association suggests that time is necessary for the relationship within the nursing system. Deliberate communication is mandated, making communication skills an important characteristic of nursing agency.

Types of Nursing Systems

There are three types of nursing systems: wholly compensatory, partly compensatory, and supportive–educative. These types can be clarified by answering one question in each nursing situation: "Who can or should perform those self-care actions . . . that require movement in space and controlled manipulation?" (Orem, 1991, p. 287). (See Figure 2.5.)

If the patient is unable to perform actions or control actions, the system is wholly compensatory; that is, the nurse performs all necessary actions. Examples include nursing systems for persons in a coma; in complete traction; or with a disease, such as severe Alzheimer's, where ambulation is possible but continuous supervision is necessary. If the nurse and patient share the responsibility for manipulative tasks and ambulation, the system is partly compensatory. Nursing systems may include those in which the patient performs most of the self-care actions related to universal requirements, but needs assistance with those related to health-deviation requirements, such as techniques required in preparation for diagnostic tests. When a patient provides all self-care requiring movement in space and controlled manipulation and the nurse performs supportive and educative action, the system is supportive-educative, or supportive-developmental. In this type of nursing system, the patient performs all self-care actions requiring ambulation and movement. For example, the nurse may provide information about breast-feeding to a new mother and support the mother psychologically during early feeding experiences. A patient

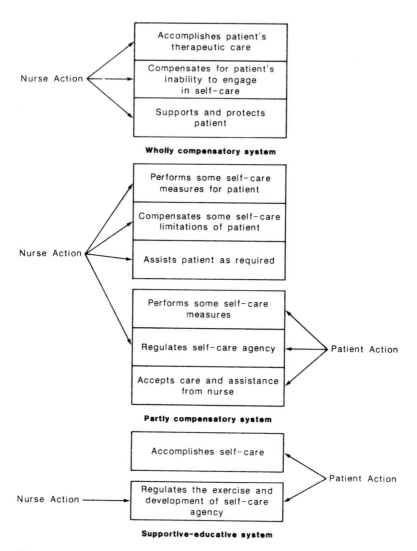

Figure 2.5. Basic nursing systems.
SOURCE: Reprinted from Orem, 1991, p. 288, by permission of Mosby-Year Book, Inc.

may need all three types of nursing systems, but at different times throughout one health condition. A patient suffering a stroke may initially need a wholly compensatory nursing system and progress to a supportive-educative nursing system. Combinations of types of systems occur at one point in time when nursing is provided to multiperson groups, such as families. The nurse may design a partly compensatory system for a home-care hospice patient and a supportive educative system for the grieving family member.

Methods of Assisting

Orem (1991) identified five general methods that persons use to assist or help others: acting for or doing for another; guiding another; supporting another, physically or psychologically; providing for a developmental environment; and teaching another (p. 286). Although these methods are not unique to nursing, they clarify the type of nursing system needed and the related roles for the nurse and patient. A grieving patient may need a supportive-educative system in which providing psychological support is the primary general method. The nurse's role is to listen in an understanding manner, while the patient's role is to actively confront and resolve a difficult situation (p. 286). Nurses tend to use the five different methods in combination within one type of nursing system. For example, a nurse may use acting and doing for to provide physical care to a post-surgical patient. Supporting another may be used to encourage the same patient to perform postoperative deep breathing and coughing exercises. Guiding another may be the general method in assisting the patient to make decisions about further medical interventions, such as chemotherapy. Teaching and providing a developmental environment may also be used within this one situation. In general, it is not appropriate to use "acting for" in the supportive-educative system. The determination of the supportive-educative system is based on the judgment that the nurse's patient is able to perform these self-care actions.

Basic Conditioning Factors

Orem (1987) describes the concept of basic conditioning factors (BCFs) as one that is peripheral to the six core, or major, concepts. It is related to two patient concepts (self-care agency and therapeutic self-care demand) and to one nurse concept (nursing agency). The basic conditioning factors, recently expanded by Orem (1991) from 8 to 10, are as follows: age, gender, developmental state, health state, sociocultural orientation, health care system elements (e.g., medical diagnosis and treatment modalities), family system elements, patterns of living, environmental factors, and resource availability and adequacy.

These factors, which are interrelated, actively influence both the quality and the quantity of self-care agency, therapeutic self-care demand, and nursing agency at instances in time. For example, age and patterns of living are BCFs that impact the universal self-care requisites of maintenance of a sufficient intake of food and water. An 18-year-old male athlete's requirements for quantity and types of nutrients and water is different from those of a 40-year-old sedentary woman. In addition, the BCFs affect self-care agency. For example, sociocultural orientation impacts a person's capability to engage in self-care. Values, folk beliefs, and practices affect the individual's self-care agency (Anna, Christensen, Hohon, Ord, & Wells, 1978; Brauch, 1985; Chamorro, 1985; Hammonds, 1985). Careful assessment of each of the BCFs is therefore necessary and serves as a critical component of the data base for determining the presence or absence of the self-care deficit. In addition, there are other factors that impact nursing agency, such as nursing education and experience (see Figure 2.1).

Propositions

A theoretical proposition is a statement that describes a concept or explains and predicts the relationship between concepts. These statements are foundational to theory and serve as the basis for theory testing and theoretical application to practice. The three types of statements are existence, definition, and relational (Walker & Avant, 1988). These serve to purport the existence of a concept, define concepts generally or theoretically, and describe the relationships among concepts, respectively. Each statement can be developed into a hypothesis for a research study. As propositions or statements are supported by research findings, the theory becomes credible and is validated. Those not supported lead to refinement or disconfirmation of the theory.

Orem's theoretical propositions are presented within the theories of self-care deficit, self-care, and nursing system. The majority of the statements further define and describe concepts in the theory. Although limited testing of propositions in the theory has been conducted (Silva, 1986), selected statements have served as the basis for research studies and will be used as examples.

Theory of Self-Care Deficit (Dependent-Care Deficit)

The first set of propositions is related to the Theory of Self-Care Deficit (or Dependent-Care Deficit) (see Table 2.2). Concepts of self-care agency (capabilities), basic conditioning factors (age, developmental state, etc.), the relationship between self-care agency and demand, a definition of the type of relationship, and nursing as a legitimate service are further described and explained through these statements. Relationships are clarified by the use of figures. For example, proposition 2 can be expressed through Figure 2.3 by examining the relationship between self-care agency and the basic conditioning factors of age, developmental state, sociocultural orientation, and health state. Because each of these factors can be considered a variable, this one proposition can become many research hypotheses. For example, Denyes (1988) studied the impact of health state on self-care ability. Health state was defined as health problems to examine the relationship between health state and self-care agency of adolescents. The significant relationship found between these two concepts provided support for proposition 2 within the theory of self-care deficit (see Table 2.2). A subsequent study by Frey and Denyes (1989) provided further support for the relationship.

Theory of Self-Care (Dependent-Care)

Six propositions within the theory of self-care provide further descriptions about the concepts of self-care and self-care system (see Table 2.2). These six propositions are a major change in the most recent edition of Orem (1991). Previously, 10 propositions provided descriptions of several concepts, including self-care requisites and dependent care (Orem, 1980; 1985b). The relationships of concepts to the basic conditioning factors were described. The revised propositions are limited to descriptions of the self-care concept, with further explanation of self-care systems and external and internal self-care actions.

Selected studies have provided initial support for Orem's earlier propositions (1980; 1985b). For example, studies by Dodd (1983, 1984a,

TABLE 2.2 Propositions in the Three Theories

Theory of Self-Care Deficit (Dependent-Care Deficit)

1. Persons who take action to provide their own self-care or care for dependents have specialized capabilities for action.

2. The individual's abilities to engage in self-care or dependent care are conditioned by age, developmental state, life experience, sociocultural orientation, health, and available resources.

3. The relationship of individuals' abilities for self-care or dependent care to the qualitative and quantitative self-care or dependent-care demand can be determined when the value of each is known.

4. The relationship between care abilities and care demand can be defined in terms of *equal to, less than, more than.*

5. Nursing is a legitimate service when:

    a. Care abilities are less than those required for meeting a known self-care demand (a deficit relationship).

    b. Self-care or dependent-care abilities exceed or are equal to those required for meeting the current self-care demand but a future deficit relationship can be foreseen because of predictable decreases in care abilities, qualitative or quantitative increases in the care demand, or both.

6. Persons with existing or projected care deficits are in, or can expect to be in, states of social dependency that legitimate a nursing relationship. (p. 71)

Theory of Self-Care (Dependent-Care)

1. Self-care is intellectualized as a human regulatory function deliberately executed with some degree of completeness and effectiveness.

2. Self-care in its concreteness is directed and deliberate action that is responsive to persons' knowing how human functioning and human development can and should be maintained within a range that is compatible with human life and personal health and well-being under existent conditions and circumstances.

3. Self-care in its concreteness involves the use of material resources and energy expenditures directed to supply materials and conditions needed for internal functioning and development and to establish and maintain essential and safe relationships with environmental factors and forces.

4. Self-care in its concreteness when externally oriented emerges as observable events resulting from performed sequences of practical actions directed by persons to themselves or their environments. Self-care that has the form of internally oriented self-controlling actions is not observable and can be known by others only by seeking subjective information. Reasons for the actions and the results being sought from them may or may not be known to the subject who performs the actions.

TABLE 2.2 Continued

5. Self-care that is performed over time can be understood (intellectualized) as an action system—a self-care system—whenever there is knowledge of the complement of different types of actions sequences or care measures performed and the connecting linkages among them.

6. Constituent components of a self-care system are sets of care measures or tasks necessary to use valid and selected means (i.e., technologies to meet existent and changing values of known self-care requisites). (pp. 69-70)

Theory of Nursing System(s)

1. Nurses relate to and interact with persons who occupy the status of nurse's patient.

2. Legitimate patients have existent and projected continuous self-care requisites.

3. Legitimate patients have existent or projected deficits for meeting their own self-care requisites.

4. Nurses determine the current and changing values of patients' continuous self-care requisites, select valid and reliable processes or technologies for meeting these requisites, and formulate the courses of action necessary for using selected processes or technologies that will meet identified self-care requisites.

5. Nurses determine the current and changing values of patients' abilities to meet their self-care requisites using specific processes or technologies.

6. Nurses estimate the potential of patients to (a) refrain from engaging in self-care for therapeutic purposes or (b) develop or refine abilities to engage in care now or in the future.

7. Nurses and patients act together to allocate the roles of each in the production of patients' self-care and in the regulation of patients' self-care capabilities.

8. The actions of nurses and the actions of patients (or nurses' actions that *compensate for the patients' action limitations*) that regulate patients' self-care capabilities and meet patients' therapeutic self-care needs constitute nursing systems. (pp. 72-73)

SOURCE: Orem (1991, pp. 69-73). Used by permission.

1984b) and Harper (1984) supported the original proposition 1, that self-care is learned behavior within the context of social groups. However, each used different populations to explore the same statement. Dodd used cancer patients receiving chemotherapy, and Harper studied black, elderly, hypertensive women attending an inner city clinic. New studies will be needed to test propositions in revised works (Orem, 1991).

Theory of Nursing System(s)

Eight propositions within the theory of nursing systems provide description of legitimate patients and nursing systems, and clarify the concept of roles for patient and nurse (see Table 2.2). Propositions 1, 4, 5, and 6 clarify the expectations for the individual in the role of nurse. Proposition 1 establishes the importance of interpersonal operations, and propositions 4 and 5 describe the methods for determining the therapeutic self-care demand and self-care agency, respectively. Propositions 2 and 3 define and describe legitimate patients; propositions 7 and 8 explain how the nurse and patient work together to determine roles and actions that become nursing systems. These propositions have served more to guide practice than as the basis for specific research studies. Taylor (1988) utilized the S-CDTN to organize and structure nursing practice, with the theory of nursing system providing structure for the nursing process. Propositions were presented and applied to the specific case study of Mr. Kay, a patient with amyotrophic lateral sclerosis, and Ms. Lee, the nurse. Proposition 7 provided clear direction to determining the roles of Mr. Kay, Ms. Lee, and others in the system before the self-care actions were assigned to any individual. Further examples of applications of research and practice are presented in Chapter 3.

Note

1. Reproduced by permission from Orem, Dorothea E., 1991, *Nursing: Concepts of practice,* 4th   ed., St. Louis: Mosby-Year Book, Inc.

3

Application to Practice, Education, and Research

The varying applications of Orem's model to practice and nursing education, as well as the utilization of the model in nursing research, are described in the following pages.

Application to Nursing Practice

The application of Orem's model to practice takes many forms in the nursing literature. For example, it has been applied to patients with specific diseases, to specific age groups, and used in a variety of settings (see Table 3.1). Each article varies in its level of application. Some authors use the model as a philosophical guide to nursing practice, often citing self-care beliefs or building on Orem's definition of self-care (e.g., Fitzgerald, 1980). Others use Orem's concepts with precision and develop guides to nursing practice (e.g. Backscheider, 1974). Many provide examples of the nursing process using a case study to develop a plan of care for an individual client (e.g. Orem & Taylor, 1986; Smith, 1989; Taylor, 1988). Applications to families have also been made (Orem, 1983a, 1983b, 1983c; Tadych, 1985; Taylor, 1989), as well as to communities (Hanchett, 1988, 1990; Orem, 1984). These applications of case examples often vary depending on the primary work used by the author. For example, Joseph (1980) presented an

TABLE 3.1 Examples of Application to Nursing Practice

Use as framework in a variety of settings:
acute care units (Mullin, 1980; Weis, 1988)
ambulatory clinics (Alford, 1985; Allison, 1973; Backscheider, 1974)
college student health program (Hedahl, 1983)
community health promotion program (Nowakowski, 1980)
critical care units (Fawcett, Cariello, Davis, Farley, Zimmaro, & Watts, 1987)
high-rise senior center (Neufeld & Hobbs, 1985)
hospices (Murphy, 1981; Walborn, 1980)
nursing homes (Anna, Christensen, Hohon, Ord, & Wells, 1978)
obstetrical units (Woolery, 1983)
pediatric units (Titus & Porter, 1989)
psychiatric units (Davidhizar & Cosgray, 1990; Moscovitz, 1984)
rehabilitation settings (Orem, 1985a)

Application to patients with specific diseases or conditions:
adolescent alcohol abusers (Michael & Sewall, 1980)
adolescents with chronic disease (McCracken, 1985)
alcoholics (Williams, 1979)
the chronically ill (Gulick, 1986)
coronary bypass surgery (Campuzano, 1982)
diabetes (Allison, 1973; Backscheider, 1974; Fitzgerald, 1980)
end stage renal disease (Michos, 1985)
enterostomies (Bromley, 1980)
head and neck surgery (Dropkin, 1981)
hypertension (Galli, 1984)
myocardial infarction (Garrett, 1985)
neurological dysfunction (Perry & Sutcliffe, 1982)
treatment with peritoneal dialysis (Perras & Zappacosta, 1982)
rheumatoid arthritis (Smith, 1989)

Application to selected age groups:
the aged (Bower & Patterson, 1986; Eliopoulos, 1984; Hankes, 1984; Hewes &
    Hannigan, 1985; Sullivan & Munroe, 1986)
children (Eichelberger, Kaufman, Rundahl, & Schwartz, 1980; Facteau, 1980;
    Koster, 1983)
mothers with newborns (Dunphy & Jackson, 1985)

overview of Orem's nursing process using Orem (1971). This edition
did not include the concept of developmental self-care requisites.
Nurses using this primary source will find variation from the current
model of nursing process described in Orem (1980, 1985b, 1991).
Taylor's (1988) work exemplifies a current application of nursing
process.

The practice literature also includes works that are modifications of Orem, such as Kinlein (1977a, 1977b) and Sullivan (1980). Chang (1980) presented a conceptual model that modified the theory for use with health care professionals promoting self-care. There are also self-care references in the nursing literature that are cited in Orem bibliographies that are not applications of Orem (e.g., Harris, 1980). The reader must distinguish between application of Orem's self-care model to practice and general application of other self-care models. Some authors combine theories or propose a blending of theoretical ideas, such as those of Orem, Leininger, and Rogers (Steiger & Lipson, 1985) and Orem and King (Swindale, 1989).

Orem's self-care model is increasingly used as a framework for practice in specific institutions. This has significant implications for nursing service administration. Newark Beth Israel Medical Center became the first acute-care hospital in the northeastern United States to base the nursing practice for the institution on Orem's model. Their library and media center are a resource for Orem's works (NLN News, 1987). Mississippi Methodist Hospital and Rehabilitation Center in Jackson, Mississippi (Allison, 1985), and Harry S Truman Hospital in Columbia, Missouri (Kunz, 1987, personal communication), have developed practical structures for implementation in their respective settings. Many Canadian health care institutions, such as those in Toronto, Scarborough, and Vancouver, use Orem's self-care theory as a model for nursing care delivery. Practical guides have been developed to facilitate implementation in their respective settings (e.g., Scarborough General Hospital, 1987). Other institutions, such as Veteran's Administration Center in Palo Alto, California, use the model on selected units. The literature is just emerging that demonstrates the effects of such application. Faucett, Ellis, Underwoood, Naqvi, and Wilson (1990) found that nurses using Orem's model differ from control nurses in their assessments and goals of care for patients in a nursing home setting.

The application to nursing service administration has been described by several authors (Miller, 1980; Nickle-Gallagher, 1985). Allison (1985) described an administrator's perspective on structuring of nursing practice based on Orem's theory of nursing. Elements of the nursing system for a patient with a spinal cord injury were developed. Self-care capabilities and limitations, self-care requisites, and related nursing actions were identified for this one patient population. Using Orem's concept of nursing agency, Allison further identified how the role and function of the professional, technical, and vocational nurse were defined in relationship to each of these components. Others (Clinton, Denyes, Goodwin, & Koto, 1977; Horn & Swain, 1977) have used Orem's concepts to develop instruments that measure patient outcomes, a method to determine the quality of nursing care.

Application to Nursing Education

Orem's framework has been used as a conceptual guide to nursing curricula in associate degree, diploma, and baccalaureate nursing programs. The number of schools currently using the model is unknown. Fawcett (1989) presented a partial listing of schools identified by Orem in personal communication. Examples included the following: Georgetown University, Washington, DC; Incarnate Word College in San Antonio; Medical College of Ohio in Toledo; Wichita State University in Wichita, Kansas; Catholic Education College in Melbourne, Australia; and Centennial College in Scarborough, Ontario. The University of Missouri-Columbia has been a leader in promoting theory development through educational and research programs. They have expanded conferences from regional to international ones in less than a decade (Eben, Gashti, Nation, Marriner-Tomey, & Nordmeyer, 1989).

The application of Orem's theory to nursing education also takes many forms. Fenner (1979) described how faculty used the model to identify curricular content that differentiated the role and function of the technical nurse from that of the professional nurse at Thornton Community College in South Holland, Illinois. Piemme and Trainor (1977) presented a rationale for exposing baccalaureate nursing students at Georgetown University to the theory early in the program. They proposed that an early understanding of Orem's theory broadened their perspective of nursing. Biehler (1987) described the development of the curricular structure at Illinois Wesleyan University in Bloomington, Illinois. The revised curriculum used seven nursing situations (Orem, 1980) to structure the clinical portion of the program. The seven disciplines of nursing knowledge identified by Orem provided an additional framework for the curricular content.

Many schools utilize Orem's nursing process in clinical practice, developing extensive assessment tools, teaching packets, and evaluation models. Herrington and Houston (1984) described the assessment tool and care plan forms used by students at the University of Southern Mississippi. The authors suggested the model and related application of Orem's process contributed to a stronger nursing focus.

The impact of a curricular structure using Orem's model is in early testing. Hartweg and Metcalfe (1986) studied the changes in self-care attitudes experienced by baccalaureate nursing students exposed to Orem's model. Using a longitudinal design, they compared attitude changes of nursing students to those of students in the general university. Self-care attitudes of nursing students increased significantly over those of general university students during the three-year period. What is not known is the impact of general nursing knowledge, not self-care knowledge, on that change. Wagnild, Rodriguez, and Pritchett (1987) surveyed nurses who had graduated from a curriculum based on Self-Care Deficit Theory of Nursing to determine if graduates used the model subsequently in their individual practice settings. Although limited by the response rate, the research suggested possible outcomes of such curricular structures, and the variables that impact the ability of graduates to apply the self-care framework in their respective clinical settings following graduation.

Utilization in Nursing Research

Orem's conceptual framework has been used increasingly as a guide for nursing research. As with practice and education, there has been much variation in the application by researchers. Some researchers use the beliefs or definitions in the model as a basis for research (e.g. Brock, & O'Sullivan, 1985). Others cite Orem's concepts, but build on the ideas of others. For example, Stollenwerk (1985) referred to supportive–educative roles of Orem, but used Gordon (1982) as a framework. Many researchers use several theories within one study (e.g., Allan, 1990). Other investigators select theoretical concepts, such as self-care or therapeutic self-care demand, to guide the research. These studies are descriptive, with a goal of describing or exploring concepts. Woods (1985) described the self-care practices of young adult married women. Kubricht (1984) used a descriptive survey to identify the therapeutic self-care demands of cancer patients having external radiation. Patterson and Hale (1985) used grounded theory to determine types of self-care practices of menstruating women.

The methods used in these studies are consistent with the recommendation of a consultant hired in the early years of the Nursing Model Committee of Catholic University (Nursing Development Conference Group, 1973). The suggestion was to refrain from using the research methods of the experimental sciences. Studies in these disciplines use precise experiments that vary one factor in a situation while holding others constant. This approach was viewed as inconsistent with Orem's model, which is based on the complexity of human systems, the patient and the nurse. The approaches recommended by the consultant were the natural history method and the hypothetical-deductive approach. The natural history approach gathers data from individuals in their natural settings, often from interviews, diaries, or through observation. Woods (1985) and Patterson and Hale (1985) are examples of this method. The hypothetical-deductive method derives hypotheses from the propositions in the theories. Recently, research using Orem's framework is appearing that uses this method for theory-testing. Harper (1984) tested four hypotheses deduced from propositions in Self-Care Deficit Theory of Nursing using a population of elderly, black, hypertensive patients. Three of these hypotheses were derived specifically from the Theory of Self-Care. The findings supported several of Orem's (1980) propositions, including the following: Self-care systems result from use of knowledge and skills to meet known requisites; and, self-care is learned within the context of social groups through human interaction and communication. Other theory-testing research continues to clarify and support the theories within the model. Hartley (1988) tested the relationship between the nursing system and self-care behavior in women learning breast self-examination. The proposition tested the relationship between a supportive–educative nursing system and self-care behavior. Frey and Denyes (1989) studied insulin dependent adolescents and found support for the relationships between universal self-care and global health state, and health deviation self-care and control of pathology. Using aggregate data on adolescents, Denyes (1988) had previously found support for distinctions between the two types of self-care. Both studies were testing the relationship between basic conditioning factors, particularly health state, and abilities to engage in self-care. Although Orem (1991) recently made changes in propositions in the theory of self-care, such testing by researchers contributes to knowledge development and further refinement of the theory.

Other investigators have not explicitly identified propositions, but have contributed to theory development by building on previous knowledge. Dodd's sequence of studies on self-care behavior of patients experiencing chemotherapy (1982, 1983, 1984a, 1984c, 1988b) and radiation therapy (1984b) included efforts to build on previous knowledge from prior studies through addressing limitations in other studies or through replication. Dodd used both descriptive (1982) and experimental (1983, 1984a) approaches. These studies supported Orem's proposition that self-care is learned within the context of social groups through human interaction and communication. Other experimental studies include Ewing (1989) with stoma patients and Williams et al. (1988) with preparation of mastectomy/hysterectomy patients. Dodd (1987; 1988a) investigated the efficacy of proactive information on self-care of radiation therapy and chemotherapy patients. However, other theories were cited in addition to Orem.

When research is conducted on theoretical concepts within a model, such as self-care agency, it is critical that a measuring instrument be valid and reliable. Much of the research within Orem's Self-Care Deficit Theory of Nursing has been directed to developing instruments to measure concepts in the model. Self-care agency is the concept most frequently operationalized by instruments. Gast et al. (1989) summarized the elements of self-care agency and described the instruments available for measurement. Other tools are in the process of development (Taylor & Geden, 1991). Jirovec and Kasno (1990) described the use of an instrument in development in both the Netherlands and the United States. The following authors have developed instruments frequently used to measure self-care agency: Denyes (1982), Hanson and Bickel (1985), and Kearney and Fleischer (1979). Kearney and Fleischer's instrument has been used to measure self-care agency of persons in East Germany (Whetstone, 1987) and Sweden (Whetstone & Hansson, 1989). Critiques and further development of the instruments have been conducted by Cleveland (1989), MacBride (1987), Riesch and Hauck (1988), and Weaver (1987). These studies are important as they raise important questions about the validity and reliability of the measurement tools. A further example of a modification of self-care agency was developed by Campbell (1986). Using Orem's framework, she developed the Danger Assessment as a measure of self-care agency of women at risk for battering.

Other investigators have developed instruments to measure self-care behaviors related to specific illnesses: side effects from cancer chemotherapy (Dodd, 1982); multiple sclerosis (Gulick, 1987); self-care medication behaviors (Harper, 1984); self-care responses to respiratory illnesses of Vietnamese (Hautman, 1987); mothers' performance of self-care for children (Moore & Gaffney, 1989); and self-care management in school-aged children with diabetes (Saucier, 1984).

Although this partial review reveals much research using Orem's model, its popularity for guiding research can be further demonstrated through a search of Dissertation Abstracts. Fawcett (1989) cited numerous examples of masters theses and dissertations that abound in the unpublished literature.

Glossary

Agency
ability, capability, or power to engage in action

Agent
the person who has the ability (agency) to perform the action or who actually performs the action

Basic conditioning factors (BCFs)
For the patient: factors that influence, at points in time, the individual's health-related needs/demands (therapeutic self-care demand) and the individual's ability (self-care agency) to engage in self-care. Examples include age, gender, health state, and family patterns.
For the nurse: factors that influence, at points, in time, the nurse's ability (nurse agency) to form interpersonal relationships and to assist with or perform self-care. Special note: In addition to the general BCFs, such nurse-specific factors as nursing experience and education also influence nursing agency.

Deliberate action
"purposeful goal- or result-seeking activity" (Orem, 1991, p. 162)

Dependent care
activities performed by responsible adults for socially dependent individuals, children, or adults to meet portions of their therapeutic self-care demands

Dependent-care agency
ability, capability, or power of a responsible adult to meet the demands
of the dependent individual

Dependent-care agent
the provider of dependent care, such as a parent, family member, or
friend. These providers can be mature adults or maturing adults, such
as adolescents.

Developmental self-care requisite
needs or goals for self-care that arise from either maturational changes
in the life cycle, such as pregnancy, or from situational events that
occur throughout human development, such as death of a significant
other

Estimative self-care operations
process of seeking knowledge about the self-care that needs to be done
(NDCG, 1979, p. 189)

Foundational capabilities and dispositions
general capabilities of self-care agency to engage in deliberate action
(NDCG, 1979)

Health
structural and functional soundness and wholeness of the individual
(Orem, 1991)

Health deviation self-care requisites
needs or goals for self-care that arise when persons are ill, injured, have
defects or disabilities, or are undergoing diagnosis or treatment

Methods of assisting
general ways of helping that can be used by one person to give
assistance to others, such as teaching, acting or doing for, guiding,
supporting, or providing for a developmental environment

Nursing agency
specialized abilities of nurses for diagnosing, prescribing, and produc-
ing nursing care that result in meeting the individual's therapeutic
self-care demand or in increasing self-care agency

Nursing system
the totality of the actions and interactions of nurses and patients and/or family in a nursing situation at a point in time

Partly compensatory nursing system
"when both nurse and patient perform care measures or other actions involving manipulative tasks or ambulation" (Orem, 1985b, p. 156)

Power components
enabling capabilities of self-care agency that must be developed and operational for individuals to perform self-care (Orem, 1987)

Productive self-care operations
process of making and doing, including the performance of the actions, monitoring the effects, and deciding to continue the actions (NDCG, 1979, p. 194)

Self-care
"practice of activities that individuals initiate and perform on their own behalf in maintaining life, health, and well-being" (Orem, 1991, p. 117)

Self-care agency
the complex, learned ability or power to perform self-care that is described as knowledge, skill, and motivation for self-care actions that promote life, health, and well-being

Self-care deficit
self-care ability of the person is not adequate to meet the therapeutic self-care demand

Self-care requisite
purposes or goals to be achieved through self-care

Supportive-educative nursing system
a nursing system in which the patient performs the actions, and the nurse guides and assists using methods of helping, such as supporting, guiding, providing for a developmental environment, and teaching. The patient is able to perform all self-care actions requiring controlled ambulation and manipulative movement.

Therapeutic self-care demand
all the self-care actions that should be performed by the individual at a point in time to maintain health and promote well-being

Transitional self-care operations
process of making judgments or decisions about what self-care should be performed; includes use of knowledge, experience, and values of the individual (NDCG, 1979, p. 194)

Universal self-care requisites
common human needs or goals of self-care that promote structural and functional integrity of the person and well-being. These include maintenance of air, food, water, and elimination; balance between activity and rest; solitude and social interaction; the prevention of hazards; and the promotion of normalcy.

Well-being
an "individual's perceived condition of existence . . . a state characterized by experiences of contentment, pleasure, and kinds of happiness; by spiritual experiences; by movement toward fulfillment of one's self-ideal; and by continuing personalization" (Orem, 1991, p. 184)

Wholly compensatory nursing system
a nursing system in which the nurse performs all the self-care actions that require controlled ambulation and manipulative movement

References

Alford, D. M. (1985). Self-care practices in ambulatory nursing clinics. In J. Riehl-Sisca (Ed.), *The science and art of self-care* (pp. 253-261). Norwalk, CT: Appleton-Century-Crofts.

Allan, J. D. (1990). Focusing on living, not dying: A naturalistic study of self-care among seropositive gay men. *Holistic Nursing Practice, 4*(2), 56-63.

Allison, S. E. (1973). A framework for nursing action in a nurse-conducted diabetic management clinic. *Journal of Nursing Administration, 3*(4), 53-73.

Allison, S. E. (1985). Structuring nursing practice based on Orem's theory of nursing: A nurse administrator's perspective. In J. Riehl-Sisca (Ed.), *The science and art of self-care* (pp. 225-235). Norwalk, CT: Appleton-Century-Crofts.

Anna, D. J., Christensen, D. G., Hohon, S. A., Ord, L., & Wells, S. R. (1978). Implementing Orem's conceptual framework. *Journal of Nursing Administration, 8*(11), 8-11.

Backscheider, J. E. (1974). Self-care requirements, self-care capabilities and nursing systems in the diabetic nurse management clinic. *American Journal of Public Health, 64*(12), 1138-1146.

Barnard, C. (1962). *The functions of the executive.* Cambridge, MA: Harvard University Press.

Biehler, B. (1987). Nursing situations as focus for curriculum design. In S. G. Taylor & E. A. Geden (Eds.), *Proceedings of the fifth annual self-care deficit theory conference: Theory-based nursing process and product using Orem's self-care theory of nursing in practice, education, research* (pp. 41-47). St. Louis, MO: Curators of the University of Missouri.

Bower, F. N., & Patterson, J. (1986). A theory-based nursing assessment of the aged. *Topics in Clinical Nursing, 8*(1), 22-32.

Brauch, M. (1985). Self-care: Black perspectives. In J. Riehl-Sisca (Ed.), *The science and art of self-care* (pp. 181-188). Norwalk, CT: Appleton-Century-Crofts.

Brock, A. M., & O'Sullivan, P. (1985). A study to determine what variables predict institutionalization of the elderly. *Journal of Advanced Nursing, 10,* 533-537.

Bromley, B. (1980). Applying Orem's self-care theory in enterostomal therapy. *American Journal of Nursing, 80,* 245-249.

Campbell, J. C. (1986). Nursing assessment for risk of homicide with battered women. *Advances in Nursing Science, 8*(4) 36-51.

Campuzano, M. (1982). Self-care following coronary artery bypass surgery. *Focus on Critical Care, 9*(2), 55-56.

Chamorro, L. C. (1985). Self-care in the Puerto Rican community. In J. Riehl-Sisca (Ed.), *The science and art of self-care* (pp. 188-195). Norwalk, CT: Appleton-Century-Crofts.

Chang, B. (1980). Evaluation of health care professionals in facilitating self-care: Review of the literature and a conceptual model. *Advances in Nursing Science, 3*(1), 43-58.

Cleveland, S. A. (1989). Re: Perceived self-care agency: A LISREL factor analysis of Bickel and Hanson's Questionnaire. [Letter to the editor]. *Nursing Research, 38, 59.*

Clinton, J. F., Denyes, M. J., Goodwin, J. O., & Koto, E. M. (1977). Developing criterion measures of nursing care: Case study of a process. *Journal of Nursing Administration 7*(7), 41-45.

Davidhizar, R., & Cosgray, R. (1990). The use of Orem's model in psychiatric rehabilitation assessment. *Rehabilitation Nursing, 15*(1), 39-41.

Denyes, M. J. (1982). Measurement of self-care agency in adolescents. *Nursing Research, 31,* 63. (Abstract)

Denyes, M. J. (1988). Orem's model used for health promotion: Directions from research. *Advances in Nursing Science, 11*(1), 13-21.

Denyes, M. J., O'Connor, N. A., Oakley, D., & Ferguson, S. (1989). Integrating nursing theory, practice, and research through collaborative practice. *Journal of Advanced Nursing, 14,* 141-145.

Dodd, M. J. (1982). Assessing patient self-care for side effects of cancer therapy: Part I. *Cancer Nursing, 5,* 447-451.

Dodd, M. J. (1983). Self-care for side effects in cancer chemotherapy: An assessment of nursing interventions: Part II. *Cancer Nursing, 6,* 63-67

Dodd, M. J. (1984a). Measuring informational intervention for chemotherapy knowledge and self-care behavior. *Research in Nursing and Health, 7,* 43-50.

Dodd, M. J. (1984b). Patterns of self-care in cancer patients receiving radiation therapy. *Oncology Nursing Forum, 11,* 23-27.

Dodd, M. J. (1984c). Self-care for patients with breast cancer to prevent side effects of chemotherapy: A concern for public health nursing. *Journal of Public Health Nursing, Dec. 1,* 202-209.

Dodd, M. J. (1987). Efficacy of proactive information on self-care of radiation therapy patients. *Patient Education, 16*(5), 538-544.

Dodd M. J. (1988a). Efficacy of proactive information on self-care in chemotherapy patients. *Patient Education and Counseling, 11,* 215-225.

Dodd, M. J. (1988b). Patterns of self-care in patients with breast cancer. *Western Journal of Nursing Research, 10,* 7-24.

Dropkin, M. J. (1981). Development of a self-care teaching program for postoperative head and neck patients. *Cancer Nursing, 4,* 103-106.

Dunphy, J., & Jackson, E. (1985). Planning nursing care for the postpartum mother and her newborn. In J. Riehl-Sisca (Ed.), *The science of art of self-care* (pp. 63-90). Norwalk, CT: Appleton-Century-Crofts.

Eben, J. D., Gashti, N. N., Nation, M. J., Marriner-Tomey, A., & Nordmeyer, S. B. (1989). Dorothea E. Orem: Self-care deficit theory of nursing. In A. Marriner-Tomey (Ed.), *Nursing theorists and their work* (2nd ed., pp. 118-132), St. Louis: C. V. Mosby.

Eichelberger, K., Kaufman, D., Rundahl, M., & Schwartz, N. (1980). Self-care nursing plan: Helping children to help themselves. *Pediatric Nursing, 6*(3), 9-13.

Eliopoulos, C. (1984). A self-care model for gerontological nursing. *Geriatric Nursing, 5*, 366-370.

Ewing, G. (1989). The nursing preparation of stoma patients for self-care. *Journal of Advanced Nursing, 14*(5), 411-420.

Facteau, L. M. (1980). Self-care concepts and the care of the hospitalized child. *Nursing Clinics of North America, 15*(1), 145-155.

Faucett, J., Ellis, V., Underwood, P., Naqvi, A., & Wilson, D. (1990). The effect of Orem's self-care model on nursing care in a nursing home setting. *Journal of Advanced Nursing, 15* 659-666.

Fawcett, J. (1989). *Analysis and evaluation of conceptual models in nursing* (2nd ed.). Philadelphia: F. A. Davis.

Fawcett, J., Cariello, F. P., Davis, D. A., Farley, J., Zimmaro, D., & Watts, R. J. (1987). Conceptual models for nursing: Application to critical care nursing practice. *Dimensions of Critical Care Nursing, 6*, 202-213.

Fenner, K. (1979). Developing a conceptual framework. *Nursing Outlook, 27*, 122-126.

Fitzgerald, S. (1980). Utilizing Orem's self-care nursing model in designing an educational program for the diabetic. *Topics in Clinical Nursing, 2*(2), 57-65.

Frey, M. A., & Denyes, M. J. (1989). Health and illness self-care in adolescents with IDDM: A test of Orem's theory. *Advances in Nursing Science, 12*(1), 67-75.

Galli, M. (1984, March/April). Promoting self-care in hypertensive clients through patient education. *Home Healthcare Nurse*, 43-45.

Garrett, A. P. (1985). A nursing system design for a patient with myocardial infarction. In J. Riehl-Sisca (Ed.), *The science and art of self-care* (pp. 142-160). Norwalk, CT: Appleton-Century-Crofts.

Gast, H. L., Denyes, M. J., Campbell, J. C., Hartweg, D. L., Schott-Baer, D., & Isenberg, M. (1989). Self-care agency: Conceptualizations and operationalizations. *Advances in Nursing Science, 12*(1), 26-38.

Gordon, M. (1982). *Manual of nursing diagnosis*. New York: McGraw-Hill.

Gulick, E. E. (1986). The self-assessment of health among the chronically ill. *Topics in Clinical Nursing, 8*(1), 74-72.

Gulick, E. E. (1987). Parsimony and model confirmation of the ADL self-care scale for multiple sclerosis persons. *Nursing Research, 36*, 278-283.

Hammonds, T. A. (1985). Self-care practices of Navajo Indians. In J. Riehl-Sisca (Ed.), *The science and art of self-care* (pp. 171-180). Norwalk, CT: Appleton-Century-Crofts.

Hanchett, E. S. (1988). Community assessment and intervention according to Orem's theory of self-care deficit. In E. S. Hanchett (Ed.), *Nursing frameworks and community as client: Bridging the gap* (pp. 25-39). Norwalk, CT: Appleton & Lange.

Hanchett, E. S. (1990). Nursing models and community as client. *Nursing Science Quarterly, 3*(2), 67-72.

Hankes, D. D. (1984). Self-care: Assessing the aged client's need for independence. *Journal of Gerontological Nursing, 10*(5), 27-31.

Hanson, B. R., & Bickel, L. (1985). Development and testing of the questionnaire on perception of self-care agency. In J. Riehl-Sisca (Ed.), *The science and art of self-care* (pp. 271-278). Norwalk, CT: Appleton-Century-Crofts.

Harper, D. C. (1984). Application of Orem's theoretical constructs to self-care medication behaviors of the elderly. *Advances in Nursing Science, 6*(3), 29-46.

Harris, J. (1980). Self-care is possible after cesarean delivery. *Nursing Clinics of North America, 15*(1), 191-204.

Harry S Truman Veteran's Administration. (1986). *Ideal sets of action for persons with laryngectomy and angina* (Columbia, MO: Unpublished work).

Hartley, L. A. (1988). Congruence between teaching and learning self-care: A pilot study. *Nursing Science Quarterly, 1*(4), 161-167.

Hartweg, D. L. (1990). Health promotion self-care within Orem's general theory of nursing. *Journal of Advanced Nursing, 15*, 35-41.

Hartweg, D. L., & Metcalfe, S. A. (1986). Self-care attitude changes of nursing students enrolled in a self-care curriculum—A longitudinal study. *Research in Nursing and Health, 9*, 347-353.

Hautman, M. A. (1987). Self-care responses to respiratory illnesses among Vietnamese. *Western Journal of Nursing Research, 9*, 223-243.

Hedahl, K. (1983). Assisting the adolescent with physical disabilities through a college health program. *Nursing Clinics of North America, 18*, 257-274.

Helene Fuld Health Trust, 1988. *The Nurse Theorists. Portraits of Excellence: Dorothea Orem* (VHS videocassette). Oakland, CA: Studio III.

Henderson, V. (1966). *The nature of nursing: A definition and its implications for practice, research, and education.* New York: Macmillan.

Herrington, J. V., & Houston, S. (1984). Using Orem's theory: A plan for all seasons. *Nursing and Health Care, 5*(1), 45-47.

Hewes, C. J., & Hannigan, E. P. (1985). Self-care model and the geriatric patient. In J. Riehl-Sisca (Ed.), *The science and art of self-care* (pp. 161-167). Norwalk, CT: Appleton-Century-Crofts.

Horn, B. J., & Swain, M. A. (1977). *Development of criterion measures of nursing care* (Vols 1-2, National Technical Information Service Nos. PB-267 004 & PB 267 005). Ann Arbor: University of Michigan.

Jirovec, M., & Kasno, J. (1990). Self-care agency as a function of patient-environmental factors among nursing home residents. *Research in Nursing and Health, 13*, 303-309.

Joseph, L. S. (1980). Self-care and the nursing process. *Nursing Clinics of North America, 15*, 131-143.

Kearney, B. Y., & Fleischer, B. J. (1979). Development of an instrument to measure the exercise of self-care agency. *Research in Nursing and Health, 2*, 25-34.

Kinlein, M. L. (1977a). *Independent nursing practice with clients.* Philadelphia: J. B. Lippincott.

Kinlein, M. L. (1977b). The self-care concept. *American Journal of Nursing, 77*, 598-601.

Koster, M. K. (1983). Self-care: Health behavior for the school-age child. *Topics in Clinical Nursing, 5*, 29-40.

Kotarbinski, T. (1965). *Praxiology: An introduction to the sciences of efficient action.* Translated from the Polish by Olgierd Wojtasiewicz (1st English ed.). New York: Pergamon Press.

Kubricht, D. W. (1984). Therapeutic self-care demands expressed by outpatients receiving external radiation therapy. *Cancer Nursing, 7,* 43-52.

Lonergan, B. J. F. (1958). *Insight: A study of human understanding.* New York: Philosophical Library.

MacBride, S. (1987). Validation of an instrument to measure exercise of self-care agency. *Research in Nursing and Health, 10,* 311-316.

Macmurray, J. (1957). *The self as agent.* London: Faber & Faber.

McCracken, M. J. (1985). A self-care approach to pediatric chronic illness. In J. Riehl-Sisca (Ed.), *The science and art of self-care* (pp. 91-104). Norwalk, CT: Appleton-Century-Crofts.

Meleis, A. I. (1985). *Theoretical nursing: Development and progress.* Philadelphia: J. B. Lippincott.

Michael, M., & Sewall, K. (1980). Use of the adolescent peer group to increase the self-care agency of adolescent alcohol abusers. *Nursing Clinics of North America, 15*(1), 157-176.

Michos, S. (1985). The application of Orem's conceptual framework to enhance self-care in a dialysis program. *American Nephrology Nurses Association Journal, 12*(1), 21-24.

Miller, J. F. (1980). The dynamic focus of nursing: A challenge to nursing administration. *Journal of Nursing Administration, 10*(1), 13-18.

Moore, J. B., & Gaffney, K. F. (1989). Development of an instrument to measure mothers' performance of self-care activities for children. *Advances in Nursing Science, 12*(1), 76-84.

Moscovitz, A. (1984). Orem's theory as applied to psychiatric nursing. *Perspectives in Psychiatric Care, 22*(1), 36-38.

Mullin, V. (1980). Implementing the self-care concept in the acute care setting. *Nursing Clinics of North America, 15*(1), 177-190.

Murphy, P. (1981). A hospice model and self-care theory. *Oncology Nursing Forum, 8*(2), 19-21.

Neufield, A., & Hobbs, H. (1985). Self-care in a high-rise for seniors. *Nursing Outlook, 33*(6), 298-301.

Nickel-Gallager, L. (1985). Structuring nursing practice based on Orem's general theory. A practitioner's perspective. In J. Riehl-Sisca (Ed.), *The science and art of self-care* (pp. 236-244). Norwalk, CT: Appleton-Century-Crofts.

NLN News. (1987). Newark Beth Israel Medical Center adopts Orem's self-care model. *Nursing & Health Care, 8*(10), 593-594.

Nowakowski, L. (1980). Health promotion/self-care programs for the community. *Topics in Clinical Nursing, 2*(2), 21-27.

Nursing Development Conference Group. (1973). *Concept formalization in nursing: Process and product.* Boston: Little, Brown.

Nursing Development Conference Group. (1979). *Concept formalization in nursing: Process and product* (2nd ed.). D. E. Orem (Ed.). Boston: Little, Brown.

Orem, D. E. (1956, October). *Hospital nursing service, an analysis.* Indianapolis: The Division of Hospital and Institutional Services, Indiana State Board of Health.

Orem, D. E. (1959). *Guides to developing curricula for the education of practical nurses.* Washington, DC: Government Printing Office. U.S. Department of Health, Education, and Welfare, Office of Education.

Orem, D. E. (1971). *Nursing: Concepts of practice.* New York: McGraw-Hill.

Orem, D. E. (1980). *Nursing: Concepts of practice* (2nd ed.). New York: McGraw-Hill.

Orem, D. E. (1983a). Analysis and application of Orem's theory. In I. W. Clements & F. B. Roberts (Eds.), *Family health: A theoretical approach to nursing care* (pp. 205-217). New York: John Wiley.

Orem, D. E. (1983b). The family coping with a medical illness. Analysis and application of Orem's self-care theory. In I. W. Clements & F. B. Roberts (Eds.), *Family health: A theoretical approach to nursing care* (pp. 385-386). New York: John Wiley.

Orem, D. E. (1983c). The family experiencing emotional crisis. Analysis and application of Orem's self-care deficit theory. In I. W. Clements & F. B. Roberts (Eds.), *Family health: A theoretical approach to nursing care* (pp. 367-368). New York: John Wiley.

Orem, D. E. (1984). Orem's conceptual model and community health nursing. In M. K. Asay & C. C. Ossler (Eds.), *Conceptual models of nursing. Applications in community health nursing. Proceedings of the Eighth Annual Community Health Nursing Conference* (pp. 35-50). Chapel Hill: Department of Public Health Nursing, School of Public Health, University of North Carolina.

Orem, D. E. (1985a). A concept of self-care for the rehabilitation client. *Rehabilitation Nursing, 10*, 33-36.

Orem, D. E. (1985b). *Nursing: Concepts of practice* (3rd ed.). New York: McGraw-Hill.

Orem, D. E. (1987). Orem's general theory of nursing. In R. Parse (Ed.), *Nursing science: Major paradigms, theories, and critiques* (pp. 67-89). Philadelphia: W. B. Saunders.

Orem, D. E. (1988). The form of nursing science. *Nursing Science Quarterly, 1*(2), 75-79.

Orem, D. E. (1988, November). *A perspective on theory based nursing.* Unpublished paper presented at the Seventh Annual Self-Care Deficit Theory of Nursing Conference, St. Louis.

Orem, D. E. (1990, September). Discussions on issues in Self-Care Deficit Theory. Remarks presented at a conference on *Self-Care Deficit Theory: Contemporary Issues,* Veterans Administration Medical Center, Palo Alto, CA.

Orem, D. E. (1991). *Nursing: Concepts of practice* (4th ed.). St. Louis: Mosby-Year Book, Inc.

Orem, D. E., & Taylor, S. G. (1986). Orem's general theory of nursing. In P. Winstead-Fry (Ed.), *Case studies in nursing theory* (Publication No. 15-2152, pp. 37-71). New York: National League for Nursing.

Parsons, T., Bales, R., & Shils, W. (1953). *Working papers in the theory of action.* Glencoe, IL: The Free Press.

Patterson, E. T., & Hale, E. S. (1985). Making sure: Integrating menstrual care practices into activities of daily living. *Advances in Nursing Science, 7*(3), 18-31.

Perras, S., & Zappacosta, A. (1982). The application of Orem's theory in promoting self-care in a peritoneal dialysis facility. *American Association of Nephrology Nurses and Technicians Journal, 9*(3), 37-39.

Perry, P., & Sutcliffe, S. (1982). Conceptual frameworks for clinical practice. *Journal of Neurosurgical Nursing, 14*(6), 318-321.

Piemme, J., & Trainor, M. (1977). A first-year nursing course in a baccalaureate program, *Nursing Outlook, 25*, 184-187.

Pridham, K. F. (1971). Instruction of a school-age child with chronic illness for increased self-care, using diabetes mellitus as an example. *International Journal of Nursing Studies, 8*, 237-246.

Riesch, S. K., & Hauck, M. R. (1988). The exercise of self-care agency: An analysis of construct and discriminant validity. *Research in Nursing & Health, 11*, 245-255.

Rosenbaum, J. N. (1989). Self-caring: Concept development for nursing. *Recent Advances in Nursing, 24*, 18-31.

Saucier, C. (1984). Self-concept and self-care management in school-age children with diabetes. *Pediatric Nursing, 10*(2), 135-138.

Scarborough General Hospital Nursing Department. (1987). *Self-care deficit theory case study guide.* Scarborough, Ontario.

Silva, M. C. (1986). Research testing nursing theory: State of the art. *Advances in Nursing Science, 9*(1), 1-11.

Smith, M.J. (1987). A critique of Orem's theory. In R.R. Parse (Ed.), *Nursing science: Major paradigms, theories, and critiques* (pp. 91-105). Philadelphia: W.B. Sanders.

Smith, M. C. (1989). An application of Orem's theory in nursing practice. *Nursing Science Quarterly, 2*(4), 159-161.

Steiger, N. J., & Lipson, J. G. (1985). *Self-care nursing. Theory & practice.* Bowie, MD: Brady Communications.

Stollenwerk, R. (1985). An emphysema client: Self-care. *Home Healthcare Nurse, 3*(2), 36-40.

Sullivan, T. (1980). Self-care model for nursing. In *Directions for nursing in the 80s* (Publication No. G-147, pp. 57-68). Kansas City: American Nurses Association.

Sullivan, T., & Munroe, D. (1986). A self-care practice theory of nursing the elderly. *Educational Gerontology, 12*, 13-26.

Swindale, J. E. (1989). The nurse's role in giving pre-operative information to reduce anxiety in patients admitted to hospital for elective minor surgery. *Journal of Advanced Nursing, 14*, 899-905.

Tadych, R. (1985). Nursing in multiperson units: The family. In J. Riehl-Sisca (Ed.), *The science and art of self-care* (pp. 49-55). Norwalk, CT: Appleton-Century-Crofts.

Taylor, S. G. (1980). *Self-Care Deficit Theory curriculum network directory.* Columbia: University of Missouri School of Nursing.

Taylor, S. G. (Ed.). (1988, November). *Nursing agency and nursing systems.* Paper presented at the Sixth Annual Self-Care Deficit Theory Conference, November 11-13, 1987, St. Louis. University of Missouri-Columbia: Curators of the University of Missouri.

Taylor, S. G. (1988). Nursing theory and nursing process: Orem's theory in practice. *Nursing Science Quarterly, 1*, 111-119.

Taylor, S. G. (1989). An interpretation of family within Orem's general theory of nursing. *Nursing Science Quarterly, 2*(3), 131-136.

Taylor, S. G. (1990, September). *Self-care deficit theory and research.* Paper presented at Self-Care Deficit Theory: Contemporary Issues. Veterans Administration Medical Center, Palo Alto, CA.

Taylor, S. G., & Geden, E. (1991). Construct and empirical validity of the self-as-carer inventory. *Nursing Research, 40*(1), 47-50.

Titus, S., & Porter, P. (1989). Orem's theory applied to pediatric residential treatment. *Pediatric Nursing, 15*(5), 465-468, 470-471, 556.

Wagnild, G., Rodriguez, W., & Pritchett, G. (1987). Orem's self-care theory: A tool for education and practice. *Journal of Nursing Education, 26*(8), 342-343.

Walborn, K. (1980). A nursing model for the hospice: Primary and self-care nursing. *Nursing Clinics of North America, 15,* 205-217.

Walker, L., & Avant, K. (1988). *Strategies for theory construction in nursing.* (2nd ed.). Norwalk, CT: Appleton & Lange.

Wallace, W. A. (1979). Basic concepts: Natural and scientific. In *From a realist point of view: Essays in the philosophy of science.* Washington, DC: University Press of America.

Wallace, W. A. (1983). Being scientific in a practice discipline. In *From a realist point of view: Essays in the philosophy of science* (2nd ed., pp. 273-293). Washington, DC: University Press of America.

Weaver, M. T. (1987). Perceived self-care agency: A LISREL factor analysis of Bickel and Hanson's questionnaire. *Nursing Research, 36,* 381-387.

Weis, A. (1988). Cooperative care and an application of Orem's self-care theory. *Patient Education Counselor, 11*(2), 141-146.

Whetstone, W. R. (1987). Perceptions of self-care in East Germany: A cross-cultural empirical investigation. *Journal of Advanced Nursing, 12,* 167-176.

Whetstone, W. R., & Hansson, A. O. (1989). Perceptions of self-care in Sweden: A cross-cultural replication. *Journal of Advanced Nursing, 14,* 962-969.

Williams, A. (1979). The student and the alcoholic patient. *Nursing Outlook, 17,* 470-472.

Williams, P., Valderrama, D., Gloria, M., Pascoguin, L., Saavedra, L., De La Rama, D., Ferry, T., Abaguin, C., & Zaldivar, S. (1988). Effects of preparation for mastectomy/hysterectomy on women's post-operative self-care behaviors. *International Journal of Nursing Studies, 25*(3), 191-206.

Woods, N. F. (1985). Self-care practices among young adult married women. *Research in Nursing and Health, 8,* 21-31.

Woolery, L. F. (1983). Self-care for the obstetrical patient: A nursing framework. *Journal of Gynecological Nursing, 12,* 33-37.

Bibliography

Classic works, articles, and chapters by Orem; critiques; comparisons with other models; and some media are presented below. Many examples of application are presented in the reference chapter. The author recognizes the significant contribution of doctoral dissertations and proceedings of conferences to theory development; they are not included below due to page constraints.

Classic Works

Nursing Development Conference Group. (1973). *Concept formalization: Process and product*. D. E. Orem (Ed.). Boston: Little, Brown.

Nursing Development Conference Group. (1979). *Concept formalization: Process and product* (2nd ed.). D. E. Orem (Ed.). Boston: Little, Brown.

Orem, D. E. (1956, October). *Hospital nursing service, an analysis*. Indianapolis: The Division of Hospital and Institutional Services, Indiana State Board of Health.

Orem, D. E. (1959) *Guides to developing curricula for the education of practical nurses*. Vocational Division No. 274, Trade and Industrial Education No. 68. Washington, DC: Government Printing Office. U.S. Department of Health, Education, and Welfare, Office of Education.

Orem, D. E. (1971). *Nursing: Concepts of practice*. New York: McGraw-Hill.

Orem, D. E. (1980). *Nursing: Concepts of practice* (2nd ed.). New York: McGraw-Hill.

Orem, D. E. (1985). *Nursing: Concepts of practice* (3rd ed.). New York: McGraw-Hill.

Orem, D. E. (1991). *Nursing: Concepts of practice* (4th ed.). St. Louis: C. V. Mosby.

Articles and Book Chapters by Orem

Orem, D. E. (1981). Nursing: a triad of action systems. In G. Lasker (Ed.), *Applied systems and cybernetics. Vol. 4. Systems research in health care, biocybernetics and ecology*. New York: Pergamon.

Orem, D. E. (1983a). The self-care deficit theory of nursing: A general theory. In I. W. Clements & F. B. Roberts (Eds.), *Family health: A theoretical approach to nursing care* (pp. 205-217). New York: John Wiley.

Orem, D. E. (1983b). The family coping with a medical illness. Analysis and application of Orem's self-care theory. In I. W. Clements & F. B. Roberts (Eds.), *Family health: A theoretical approach to nursing care* (pp. 385-386). New York: John Wiley.

Orem, D. E. (1983c). The family experiencing emotional crisis. Analysis and application of Orem's self-care deficit theory. In I. W. Clements & F. B. Roberts (Eds.), *Family health: A theoretical approach to nursing care* (pp. 367-368). New York: John Wiley.

Orem, D. E. (1984). Orem's conceptual model and community health nursing. In M. K. Asay & C. C. Ossler (Eds.), *Conceptual models of nursing. Applications in community health nursing. Proceedings of the Eighth Annual Community Health Nursing Conference* (pp. 35-50). Chapel Hill: Department of Public Health Nursing, School of Public Health, University of North Carolina.

Orem, D. E. (1985). A concept of self-care for the rehabilitation client. *Rehabilitation Nursing, 10*(3), 33-36.

Orem, D. E. (1987). Orem's general theory of nursing. In R. Parse (Ed.), *Nursing science: Major paradigms, theories, and critiques* (pp. 67-89). Philadelphia: W. B. Saunders.

Orem, D. E. (1988). The form of nursing science. *Nursing Science Quarterly, 1*(2), 75-79.

Orem, D. E. (1989). Theories and hypotheses for nursing administration. In B. Henry, C. Arndt, M. DiVincenti, & A. Marriner-Tomey (Eds.), *Dimensions of nursing administration*. Boston: Blackwell Scientific.

Orem, D. E., & Taylor, S. G. (1986). Orem's general theory of nursing. In P. Winstead-Fry (Ed.), *Case studies in nursing theory* (Publication No. 15-2152, pp. 37-71). New York: National League for Nursing.

Analyses and Critiques of Self-Care Deficit Theory of Nursing

Dashiff, C. J. (1988). Theory development in psychiatric-mental health nursing: An analysis of Orem's theory. *Archives of Psychiatric Nursing, 11*, 366-372.

Davidhizar, R. (1989). Critique of Orem's self-care model. *Nursing Management, 19*(11), 78-79.

Eben, J. D., Gashti, N. N., Nation, M. J., Marriner-Tomey, A., & Nordmeyer, S. B. (1989). Dorothea E. Orem: Self-care deficit theory of nursing. In A. Marriner-Tomey (Ed.), *Nursing theorists and their work* (2nd ed., pp. 118-132), St. Louis: C. V. Mosby.

Fawcett, J. (1989). *Analysis and evaluation of conceptual models in nursing* (2nd ed.). Philadelphia: F. A. Davis.

Johnston, R. L. (1989). Orem's self-care model of nursing. In J. Fitzpatrick & A. Whall (Eds.), *Conceptual models of nursing: Analysis and application* (2nd ed., pp. 165-184). Norwalk, CT: Appleton & Lange.

Foster, P. C., & Janssens, N. P. (1985). Dorothea E. Orem. In Nursing Theories Conference Group, *Nursing theories: The base for professional nursing practice* (2nd ed., pp. 124-139). Englewood Cliffs, NJ: Prentice-Hall.

Meleis, A. I. (1985). *Theoretical nursing: Development and progress.* Philadelphia: J. B. Lippincott.

Meleis, A. I. (1991). *Theoretical nursing: Development and progress* (2nd ed.). Philadelphia: J. B. Lippincott.

Melynk, K. A. M. (1983). The process of theory analysis: An examination of the nursing theory of Dorothea E. Orem. *Nursing Research, 32,* 170-174. [Letters to the editor and responses by the author, *Nursing Research, 32,* 318; 381-383.]

Lundh, U., Soder, M., & Waerness, K. (1988). Nursing theories: A critical view. *IMAGE: Journal of Nursing Scholarship, 20*(1), 36-40.

Smith, M. C. (1979). Proposed metaparadigm for nursing research and theory development. An analysis of Orem's self-care theory. *IMAGE: The Journal of Nursing Scholarship, 11,* 75-79.

Smith, M. J. (1987). A critique of Orem's theory. In R. R. Parse (Ed.), *Nursing science: Major paradigms, theories, and critiques* (pp. 91-105). Philadelphia: W. B. Saunders.

Stevens, B. J. (1984). *Nursing theory: Analysis, application, and evaluation. (2nd ed.).* Boston: Little, Brown.

Thibodeau, J. A. (1983). *Nursing models: Analysis and evaluation.* Monterey, CA: Wadsworth Health Science Division.

Whelan, E. G. (1984). Analysis and application of Dorothea Orem's self-care practice model. *Journal of Nursing Education, 23*(8), 342-345.

Media and Software

Helene Fuld Health Trust, 1988. *The Nurse Theorists. Portraits of Excellence: Dorothea Orem* (VHS videocassette). Oakland, CA: Studio III.

National League for Nursing. (1987). *Nursing theory: A circle of knowledge.* New York: Author.

Orem, D. E. (1978, December). *A general theory of nursing* [Audio cassette recording]. Paper presented at the Second Annual Nurse Educator Conference, New York.

Self-care deficit theory of nursing: Software for bedside care [computer program]. Bordentown, NJ: Nursing Systems International.

Comparisons With Self-Care Models and Nursing Models

Butterfield, S. (1983). In search of commonalities: An analysis of two theoretical frameworks. *International Journal of Nursing Studies, 20,* 15-22.

Gantz, S. B. (1990). Self-care: Perspectives from six disciplines. *Holistic Nursing Practice, 4*(2), 1-12.

Hanucharurnkul, S. (1989). Comparative analysis of Orem's and King's theories. *Journal of Advanced Nursing, 14*, 365-372.

Rosenbaum, J. (1986). Comparison of two theorists: Orem and Leininger. *Journal of Advanced Nursing, 11*, 409-419.

Steiger, N. J., & Lipson, J. G. (1985). *Self-care nursing. Theory & practice*. Bowie, MD: Brady Communications.

Woods, N. F. (1989). Conceptualizations of self-care: Toward health-oriented models. *Advances in Nursing Science, 12*(1), 1-13.

About the Author

Donna L. Hartweg is an Associate Professor and Director, School of Nursing, Illinois Wesleyan University, Bloomington, IL, where she has taught in the Orem guided curriculum for over 10 years. She has presented at national and international conferences on Self-Care Deficit Theory of nursing and is author and coauthor of several self-care articles. Her most recent work is on Health Promotion Self-Care within Orem's general theory of nursing, published in the *Journal of Advanced Nursing*. Her current research is on the health promotion self-care practices of healthy middle-aged women. Throughout her doctoral studies at the College of Nursing, Wayne State University, Detroit, she was active in the Orem Research Group.